CONTENTS

CONTENTS

WHY A NATIONAL HEALTH SERVICE?

WHY A NATIONAL HEALTH SERVICE?

the part played by the Socialist Medical
Association

D. Stark Murray

PEMBERTON BOOKS

First published 1971 by Pemberton Books
(Pemberton Publishing Co Ltd), 88 Islington
High Street, London N1 8EN

ISBN 0 301 71121 6 *cloth*
     0 301 71122 4 *paper*

Printed in Great Britain by
Richard Clay (The Chaucer Press) Ltd
Bungay, Suffolk

INTRODUCTION

The year 1970 was the fortieth year of the Socialist Medical Association which has had a unique political history that seems worthy of some detailed study. The SMA was founded in 1930 for one purpose, the introduction of a national health service based on socialist principles: saw its ideas carried into effect in eighteen years and so is able in its fortieth year to look back not only at the initial struggle and success but to assess after another twenty-one years, the success of the National Health Service.

The band of doctors and other health workers who formed the SMA varied in their political views and might have opposed each other on some political issues but in fact never had a 'split' but remained steadfast in pursuit of one idea. From time to time diversionary movements may have attracted a few members but the members as a whole never wavered in their programme: and never had any doubt that they would achieve it by and through the Labour Party. They gained great strength over the years from the support of the whole Labour movement and from the recognition among its leaders that health had to have top priority.

Today's members turn with pleasure to the verdict of an American historian, Almont Lindsey, given in his book, *Socialised Medicine*, that the 'British National

Health Service must be regarded as one of the great achievements of the twentieth century'. That pleasure is not one of complacency for the SMA knows that the health service will be protected, developed and improved only by as resolute a struggle in the remaining thirty years of the century as in the previous forty.

ONE

THE EARLY BEGINNINGS

Why has Great Britain a National Health Service, and why is it firmly based on socialist principles? The short answer is because there came into existence at a crucial political moment, a Socialist Medical Association; the longer answer lies in the history of medico-political thought which led to the examination of certain principles of medical service which could be realized only in socialist political action. Medicine and the way in which medical attention is given have been evolving for a very long time but whenever a doctor–philosopher sat down to think of the best way of attending to the health and the illnesses of mankind, he reached similar conclusions. Allowing for the vastly different circumstances, Hippocrates, 2,400 years ago, was saying the same as the SMA was to say in 1930, as Aneurin Bevan and a Labour Government were to say in 1946. All declared that the physician should do his work without any reference to the social, financial or racial position of the patient and that the necessary medical attention, preventive or curative, should be given without any question of fees arising.

The National Health Service Act crystallizes in legal language what the SMA had said was necessary, that the service should be preventive, curative and educative, that it should be universally available. These are monumental principles departing completely from the language of free enterprise, self-seeking and un-principled money-making which are the mark of capitalist society. Insofar as they have not been completely translated into action and services we are still short of the ideal, but the foundations for further evolution have been soundly based.

These principles are soundly based both medically and politically. Medically they 'take medicine out of the market place' and elevate it to a social service in which the skilled doctor can apply all his knowledge to the care of both the individual patient and the community without any reference to cost, or the financial and social standing of the sick person. For the doctor who has any sense of vocation this is a great freedom far above all other freedoms to which he might aspire, and places the physician or surgeon in a unique position exceeded only by his unique part in matters of life and death.

Politically these principles are those of socialism and so set the scene for the next step to a socialist society. They placed upon a Minister of Health, answerable to Parliament and so to the people, the responsibility for the quantity and quality of services to be supplied. It was to be comprehensive and available to all citizens and so, by implication, of top quality: and was to provide for the prevention of disease, for the treatment of all diseases, for rehabilitation and for the education of the people in matters of health. It was to be paid for out of general national income although for a time part of the cost was to be met from the weekly contributions of those in employment.

To reach these conclusions and to translate them into legislation had been a long process. The whole nineteenth century was occupied with slow moves away from all the horrors and disease associated with the poverty and degradation of child labour, of long working hours, of intense hardship in factories and mines.

In the second half of the century the discovery of the part played by bacteria in disease, especially typhoid, cholera and tuberculosis led to further schemes to control such conditions.

What is seldom noticed is how large a part the combination of disease with poverty played in the origins and growth of the Labour Movement which was to culminate in the National Health Service. From Robert Owen through Keir Hardie to Beatrice and Sydney Webb and on to Aneurin Bevan, the ill health associated with working class poverty was a great spur to the development of their socialist views. Hardie indeed saw socialism as the cure for the physical ills of his own class as well as the basic faults of capitalism and the British Labour Party's origin lies in this and not in Marxist or other economic theories. By the beginning of this century we had made a start on public health measures but the Webbs clearly stated that this was not enough: a state medical service would be essential to establish a healthy nation.

Health has been a subject much discussed down the ages and attempts to provide medical care had been made in many places at various times. The Churches had played a very big part in providing some kind of charity for the poor leading to poor-law systems in many countries. By the middle of the nineteenth century the great political minds began to cogitate on the subject and writers began to put forward new ideas. Samuel Butler in *Erewhon* shocked many Victorians into asking if health was a right or a duty, if illness was a departure from duty or an act of God; and if medical care was to be regarded as a privilege or something to be denied to those wicked enough to become ill.

In most utopian writings health was assumed to be inherent in citizens of a properly organized society and in *News from Nowhere* everyone appears to abound in health. Edward Bellamy, in *Looking Backward*, however, thought that even in Utopia they would still have the sick, the crippled, the disabled and the blind, and speaking of the year AD 2000 said that 'those who cannot work are conceded the full right to live on the produce of those who can'. He saw with astonishing clarity the principle of universality of services. 'A solution which leaves an unaccounted-for residuum is no solution at all. Our resolution of the problem of human society would have been none at all had it left the lame, the sick, and the blind outside with the beasts to fare as they might.'

Bellamy, writing in 1887, saw clearly that not only should health be a human right but that a medical service would have to be organized by the State. He rejected the idea of a bureaucratic and impersonal service which he thought would not create the proper and desirable doctor–patient relationship. 'The good a physician can do a patient depends largely on his acquaintance with his constitutional tendencies and conditions. The patient must be able, therefore, to call in a particular doctor, and he does so, just as patients in your day.' He is, of course, speaking to an 1887 traveller who has arrived in AD 2000 with a very inquiring mind. 'The only difference is that, instead of collecting a fee for himself, the doctor collects it for the nation by ticking off the amount from the patient's credit card.' (Bellamy not only invented credit cards but prophesied radio.) His book became the bible of many reformers and as it coincided with the great public health developments that were just beginning, put health in the forefront of political discussions.

It was, however, the early Fabians who first made health a truly political subject and it was the Minority

Report on the Poor-Law (1909) signed by Mrs Webb, George Lansbury and two other members (but generally attributed in large measure to Sydney Webb) that first spelled out the need for the first principles of 'a State medical service'. The principles of such a service would lead 'in practice as well as in theory, to searching out disease, securing the earliest possible diagnosis, taking hold of the incipient case, removing injurious conditions, applying specialized treatment, enforcing healthy surroundings and personal hygiene, and aiming always at preventing either recurrence or spread of disease in contrast to the mere "relief" of the individual'. At that moment even the Webbs and George Lansbury did not see how they could insist on a free service for all but they demanded 'a unified service on public health lines'. 'It is clear,' they went on, 'that in the public interest neither the promptitude nor the efficiency of the medical treatment must be in any way limited by considerations of whether the patient can or should repay its cost.'

After the beginning of the twentieth century it was of course the rising tide of the political Labour movement and of the trade unions that forced Lloyd George to introduce the National Health Insurance system in 1911. Such a concept had no place in his basic political thinking at that date but the trade union demand for better conditions included the need for some form of medical care, at least for those in work which at that time meant mainly men, except in a few industries. This was finally accepted, but only for those of low income.

That system of Health Insurance, providing general practitioner care and drugs for those paying their weekly stamps was to last until 1948. But it was seen by pioneers in the medical profession to be quite inadequate; and indeed the principles of today's health service were already clearly stated before the NHI Act became law. Most people who write about health services are completely ignorant of the exact and continuous line from these pioneers through to the National Health Service. There were many false trails and side-tracking movements but the writings of a handful of men around 1910–14 were the real origin of all that is now important in health services. In 1910 Benjamin Moore, a Liverpool physician, could write, in *The Dawn of the Health Age*, 'Now there is a great and general awakening of the public mind, voiced by the thoughts and actions of millions of the best of the inhabitants of the country, toward a real scientific and continued endeavour to deal with the problems of poverty and disease in a way that means eradication from the race and not merely amelioration of the lot of the individual.' He was probably the first to use the words National Health Service, the construction of which 'is a process which will require a generation for its completion and the collaboration of many active minds of skilful administrators'.

So he demanded a service which was national in structure, preventive and curative, in which all doctors would be salaried in a 'unified system of hospitals and doctors no longer in deadly opposition to one another but working for a common cause, in short a modern machine and weapon of warfare against disease, instead of a fragmentary and motley museum of survivals from antiquity'. GPs would service between 460 and 500 families and surgeries would be run on an appointment system, 'no crowds, no sweated work'; the GP would 'have no rivals, no bills to bother about . . . free from a hundred embarrassments in his work from which he now suffers'. He saw no division but rather complete cooperation between the GP, the hospital doctor, the public health officer and sanitary inspector to get rid of all infectious disease.

There is scarcely an item of disease prevention or form of medical care which we argue about today which Dr Benjamin Moore did not discuss. He wanted a preventive health service for, he said, 'more care is bestowed by the law upon the succulency of oysters than upon the safety of the human beings who eat them'. He wanted a proper occupational health service for 'disease is secondary to the calls of industry and commerce; the overcrowding and insanitary conditions in many workshops are a dishonour in face of our knowledge as well as a constant menace to life and to health'. He demanded, in 1913, that 'disease should be made a *primary* consideration in the country and the Health Service should be under the care of a Cabinet Minister directly responsible to Parliament and people for the maintenance of health and proper control of disease'. But it is small wonder he got little support for he actually thought a Minister of Health should 'possess professional and technical knowledge of his subject'.

The medical profession as a whole did not listen to Benjamin Moore, especially when he spoke of the wonderful effects of a salaried service—'Book-keeping, debt collections and bad debts would have vanished like an evil dream, and the doctor would at last feel that he was an honoured member of a scientific profession, with time and interest to study the problems which he had chosen for his life work, instead of being, as he is now, *a small tradesman with a declining business.*' But he influenced many including Dr H. H. Mac-William, then beginning his career at Walton Hospital, from which twenty years later was to come *The Walton Plan* for a hospital service. However, so many people did support Dr Moore that he was able to establish the State Medical Service Association which held its first meeting on July 26, 1912, and continued to exist, with varying fortunes and activities until it was replaced by the Socialist Medical Association in 1930. But the line of thought was continuous, for among those who were active in both associations was Somerville Hastings to whom the Labour Party owed more than it has ever acknowledged for the working out of a practical health service. However, it is worth recalling what the State Medical Service Association said at its inaugural meeting. Among other things, the basis of the programme was to include:

1. The whole profession to be organized on the lines of other State Services now in existence.
2. Entry to the profession to be by one State examination.
3. Each member of the Service to be paid an adequate salary, increasing gradually according to length of service and position in the service and to be entitled to a pension.
4. Members of the public to have as far as possible *free choice of doctor*: but no doctor to be called upon to have charge of more than a specified number of patients.
5. The service to be preventive and curative; all hospitals to be nationalized and used for the purposes of consultative, operative and therapeutic work *at the request and in conjunction with the patient's own doctor*.
6. The service to be open to every man, woman and child—rich or poor.

By October of the same year 135 doctors had joined the State Medical Service Association and meetings were held all over the country, deputations were sent to see the Prime Minister and others: and invitations, of which few were accepted, to be Vice-Presidents were sent to prominent people including such political opposites as Arthur Balfour, Ramsay MacDonald, Neville Chamberlain, Mrs M. G. Fawcett, George Barnes, Donald MacAlister, Oliver Lodge, W. A. Appleton and Arthur Henderson.

The State Medical Service Association was fortunate in having among its members many who were ready with the pen. Dr Charles A. Parker acted as Secretary for a time and contributed articles to many journals and two of these were reprinted from *The Medical World* as a pamphlet in the autumn of 1912. He was one of the first to draw attention to the bad distribution of doctors and to relate that to death rates. Hampstead had one doctor to 476 people, a birth rate of 14 per 1,000, an infantile death rate of 60 and a death rate from infectious diseases of 0·56; Walsall had one doctor to 2,096 people, a birth rate of 29, an infantile death rate of 133 and a death rate from infectious diseases of 1·52. Bermondsey was another example with corresponding figures of one doctor to 4,065, birth rate 31, infantile deaths 157 and infectious disease death rate 3·93. No wonder he demanded that the salaries paid to doctors in Bermondsey 'must certainly be as good as those paid in Hampstead and possibly better'.

To get better distribution of doctors he wanted the population divided into units of 100,000 with its hospital as the centre of all medical care but all GPs 'as essential a part of the staff of the hospital as are consultants'—and all Medical Officers of Health to have their headquarters in the same building as all other doctors. But all doctors would also work at 'receiving stations' well equipped with instruments and all modern appliances. Each 100,000 unit would, he estimated, need 86 doctors, six resident in a 200-bed hospital and 50 GPs of various grades. The 80 non residents would then cost £36,000 a year! The cost to the nation would have been £24½ million. Those who find it difficult to calculate how many doctors we need today would be interested in Dr Charles Parker's figures:

Consultants and specialists	12,150
Resident Medical Officers	2,430
General Practitioners	20,250
	34,850

What a service that number, organized in such a way, could have given to the population of that date, 40½ millions.

These early reformers were quickly labelled 'socialists' and one Dr R. T. Irving of Southport went to great lengths to explain and discuss the term. He considered the British Medical Association's views to be 'unbusinesslike, impolitic contentions—they are never unselfish, they demand much from the public and guarantee no better service in return'. He thought 'a National Medical Service is socialistic; it is an attempt to better health and life that the individual may more readily assert himself'. He wanted less money for his service than Dr Parker but did not set out his ideas so clearly.

Clearest of all was Dr Milson Rupert Rhodes of Didsbury, Manchester. A pamphlet based on an address he gave in 1912 to the BMA in Manchester is dedicated 'to my fellow workers in our beloved profession, who, in the BMA, in the National Medical Union and in all other societies, are united in the cause of Medical efficiency and the public good'. He took the headings of the State Medical Service Association quoted above and extended them in the greatest detail.

He did not use the words Health Centre and he thought of every doctor having access to hospital beds, and so he asked for a 'central depot to be instituted in every locality'; doctors in the neighbourhood were to act as the management committee although the facilities were to be provided by Government. The central depot, he declared, 'will thus be in the nature of:

1. A cottage hospital.
2. A centre of scientific work in the locality.
3. A nursing home.
4. A board room for doctors.
5. A medical library and
6. A central supply depot both for sterile instruments, sera, laboratory equipment and therapeutic apparatus.'

He visualized that while most patients would get surgical treatment free there would be some 'of the poor middle class, never yet provided for'—who could get operations done at a moderate fixed tariff since surgeons would 'not require the great fees of the present day as they will receive proper remuneration for their hospital work'. He did not advocate, as some of his colleagues did, a complete salaried service, but was obviously trying to find a compromise which would provide a national service with some place for modified private practice. He thought Manchester should give a lead to the rest of the country and quoted with approval from a Manchester pamphlet of 1889 in which a Dr Rentoul had proposed the formation of a Public Medical Service which the doctors refused 'because they thought it would affect their money interests'. Dr Rhodes believed the medical profession were wrong then and should, in 1912, see that a national service would release doctors 'from all base and degrading advertising expediencies, from flunkyism and all that is mean and unmanly'.

The Minute Book of the State Medical Service Association is fascinating reading. Sydney Webb gave an address on the need for and possible structure of a Board of Health. He was quite emphatic on a point that was to crop up again in 1946, that doctors should not be members of governing committees but should work through advisory committees. He and others had, of course, no doubt the medical administrators would have a very important place and that management committees should be small. The SMSA met regularly and all through World War I continued its work, discussed its relations with the rising Labour Party and continuously advocated the setting up of a Ministry of Health as a preliminary step to a national medical service.

It must indeed have been a great effort to keep such a highly specialized organization going during war time and yet the executive met seventeen times during that period. Many members resigned because of war service or because they could not afford the fee but the EC retained their names on the membership list. Mr Somerville Hastings appears to have assumed as early as February 1915 the job he continued to do for the next forty years 'drafting a circular to go out to all members' and at the same time giving unparalleled leadership.

The annual subscription was fixed at 2/6d and every member was to get 'such literature as the Association might publish'. Because of travel difficulties a small committee of London members was given executive powers.

As was to happen again in World War II, the impact of war made many members of the medical profession ask what was to happen when peace returned. It is said that two factors inclined many toward a salaried service, their war time experience of such a service and the fact that incomes were very low. Much discussion took place 'more pronounced in Lancashire and the North than in the South'. At its meeting on April 19, 1917, twelve members considered two draft plans for a State medical service and it was decided to seek an interview with the President of the Local Government Board and to press on him the urgency of setting up a Ministry of Health. That the subject was becoming one of importance is shown by the publication by the *Lancet* in its issue of July 20, 1918, of three lengthy articles on the post war reconstruction of the medical services. All foresaw changes, particularly the article of Sir Bernard (later Lord) Dawson which was to be further elaborated in a Ministry of Health 'Consultative Council' report two years later. The indefatigable Drs Moore and Parker gave the arguments for a salaried unified health service, and this time pressed the need for group practice at 'clinical centres'. They visualized all health workers working together and said 'the work of the clinical service would centre around the hospitals or treatment centres in close touch with the hospitals and *general practitioners would share the clinical work and form an integral part of the staff of the hospitals. They would work in groups.*'

The *Lancet* wrote a leader on the articles it had published and summarized its own views in a very forward looking way. 'There appears to be no doubt in the public as well as the professional mind that now is the appointed time for placing the medical profession on a more stable basis, both as a calling for its members and as a service whereby the health of the people is to be maintained by the best preventive and curative measures.' If not all was done that could have been done at least a Ministry of Health was established and had a physician, Dr Christopher Addison, as its first Minister. He at once set up a Consultative Council on Medical and Allied Services with Lord Dawson of Penn as its Chairman and its first task was to consider the kind of scheme necessary to provide 'such forms of medical and allied services as should be available for the inhabitants of a given area'.

When this body quickly presented an interim report because it felt the matter was urgent, and when it accepted that 'the general availability of services can only be effected by new and extended organization, *distributed according to the needs of the community*', and when it recommended Health Centres as the SMSA had been pressing for ten years, that body suffered a typical setback, some of its members thinking the job was finished and failing to realize just how long a battle still had to be fought before the Health Centres would be built. The Dawson Report is often spoken of as if it invented Health Centres but as we have shown this is far from true. It did accept the basic principle that 'the best means of maintaining health and curing disease should *be made available to all citizens*'. It spoke as if the work of the SMSA had already established the concept of the Health Centre for it said 'A Health Centre *is* an institution wherein are brought together various medical services, preventive and curative, so as to form one organization.' But the Dawson Report shows no inkling of group practice and its Primary Health Centres were a combination of a cottage hospital with plenty of private pay-beds and a clinic, and the GP was to be left to decide which of his patients would be seen in his own surgery or at the health centre. The Secondary Health Centres were an ill conceived attempt to bring some kind of organization into the hospital service but never found favour. As to the main plank of the SMSA, whole time salaried service, the Dawson Report adhered to the profession's reactionary view that 'by its adoption the public would be serious losers . . . whole time salaried service would tend by its machinery to discourage initiative, to diminish the sense of responsibility and to encourage mediocrity'. A strange reaction so soon after a war in which surgery in the hands of whole time officers had made great advances. As it turned out, political changes and post war problems drove the health service question into the background.

It was not surprising, therefore, that the membership of the SMSA fell, although Dr Charles Parker continued as Secretary. It was the work of a few new members, Mr Somerville Hastings, Dr Lyster (a medical officer of health), Alfred Salter, later MP for Bermondsey, and Dr Hector Munro who was still doing propaganda thirty years later, which kept the movement alive. Meetings tended to be small and infrequent although the same names continued to appear in the historic minute book. Dr Jane Walker, a real pioneer among women physicians, acted as Chairman and then as Treasurer, but Mr Somerville Hastings with his friend Dr Lawson Dodd were most active inside the Labour Party. Indeed the members of the executive committee were busy also in the Fabian Society and as an advisory committee on health matters to the Labour Party.

When next the SMSA becomes reactivated it is December 1929 and new names have joined the few older ones still left. Mr Hastings has taken the place of Professor Moore as leader and is supported by Drs Ethel Stacey, Victor Patterson, Robert Forgan, Oscar Tobin, Arnold Sorsby; Dr John MacKeith, and Dr H. Billing among the twenty-six members who attended the meeting. Much discussion took place on whether the association was to be connected with the Labour Party and it was decided it should be 'non-party' and its name changed to National Medical Service Association.

Its views on policy were however an advance on those we have quoted from earlier pamphlets and very close to those which very shortly were to become clearly political aims achievable only through the Labour Party. The Association was to advocate:

1. A free National Medical Service available to all members of the community and providing every form of medical, surgical, obstetrical, dental and preventive treatment.
2. The provision of necessary institutional treatment, consultant and specialist services including bacteriological, pathological and X-ray, together with all known means for the treatment and prevention of disease.
3. All to be coordinated in one service by the Ministry of Health.

There seems to have been no difference on these points as basic principles but there developed quite sharp divisions of opinion as to how they were to be attained. Dr Alfred Salter was particularly keen to make a step toward a national service through the extension of the existing health insurance scheme. He told a meeting that the quickest advance would be by extending health insurance to all dependents of workers for British democracy always advances 'by stages and by grafting on to existing schemes'. But it would be essential to get the scheme under the control of the Ministry of Health and the local authorities instead of existing insurance committees. That was, in fact, the view of the Public Health Advisory Committee of the Labour Party. The general political atmosphere was so much in favour of such an advance that Dr Salter told the meeting that it would be presented to Parliament as soon as time could be found. Dr Salter could not guess it would be seventeen years before a Minister of Health could persuade Parliament to consider a National Health Service Bill.

A year later in 1930, the National Medical Service Association met for the last time. One subject discussed was whether it should amalgamate with the newly formed Socialist Medical Association but it was decided there was a place for both organizations. Events were to prove that there was no place for both and it was the more definitely political and much younger body, the Socialist Medical Association that was to survive. That this was so was probably largely due to the decision of Mr Somerville Hastings to accept nomination as President of the SMA, a position he occupied for twenty years. During the whole of that time, as we shall see, he kept up the continuous propaganda for a fully developed national health service which he had already been advocating since the end of World War I.

Public opinion was rapidly accepting the idea of a national medical service and in a way Somerville Hastings in lectures and articles to journals reflected this very accurately, since he maintained the closest contact with the people in his constituency, at that time, Reading. In 1928, the *Lancet* printed an article by him on 'The Future of Medical Practice in England' which was very tentative but based on a firm belief in the inevitability of 'the provision by the State of some form of public medical service within the next few years'. Lay audiences, he wrote, always applauded the idea and he called on the medical profession to begin planning such a service instead of leaving it to others whose scheme might 'be ill digested and imperfect'. As a specialist, it is interesting to note Hastings fully appreciated the need for a scheme in which 'the general practitioner may have an honoured place as the natural centre around which the whole scheme revolves'.

Three years later, on May 10, 1931, Somerville Hastings gave the first Presidential address to the Annual Meeting of the Socialist Medical Association, setting out in his first sentence the role of that body. 'It is the privilege of a new organization to see visions and dream dreams but in looking into the future we must be strictly practical.' His basic principles for a new type of medical service were that it should be preventive, that 'there must be no economic barrier between doctor and patient', that all citizens should have a right to hospital care, that the team and not the individual should be the keynote but in that team 'the general practitioner is essential'. The President told the SMA that such a service, guaranteeing choice of doctor and professional freedom, should operate from medical centres which ideally would also house the dental service, would have visits from hospital consultants and provide a basic industrial health service. It was in this speech that one brand new and important concept, that 'specialists attached to the hospitals would also consult with the members of the general practitioner service in the patients' homes', first appeared. It was from this moment, indeed, that a great variety of thoughts on how a health service can best be provided began to come together and to make a cohesive whole but one of that 'practical nature' which was to appeal to the Labour Party and ultimately to the whole nation.

TWO

THE SOCIALIST MEDICAL ASSOCIATION

SOCIALIST THINKERS in Germany and Austria were a little ahead of their British contemporaries in preparing schemes for basic medical treatment services and it was from one of these, a Dr Ewald Fabian who practised dentistry in Berlin, that a direct stimulus to form a socialist organization came. What has been said about the National Medical Service Association indicates that the political need was already clear to some but had not crystallized in an actual organization. Early in the summer of 1930 Dr Charles Brook, as he tells in *Making Medical History*, received a letter from Dr Fabian telling him that there already existed in many European countries 'organizations of Socialist members of the medical profession'. The German organization already had several hundred members and published its own journal *Der Sozialistiche Arzt* (The Socialist Doctor). Dr Fabian edited this journal and wrote to express his surprise that there was no British organization with which he could exchange ideas. Dr Brook's name had attracted his attention through a report of a speech made at a London County Council meeting. Dr Brook was fighting for better amenities in Tooting, a constituency which he fought in a Parliamentary election and was at first reluctant to take on other work but was finally persuaded by Dr Fabian. (He was later forced to leave Germany and died in New York in 1946.) This part of the story has already been told by Dr Charles W. Brook in *Making Medical History* which he published in 1946 and from this one quotes at some length. Although Dr Fabian had persuaded Dr Brook of the need for a new organization it was annoyance at a speech by Sir Ernest Graham-Little, MD, then Independent MP for London University, that gave the final stimulus. Graham-Little was a bitter opponent of any step toward a State medical service and a speech he made at this time triggered off the formation of the Socialist Medical Association. Dr Brook wrote to the *Daily Herald*, 'inviting medical practitioners who might be interested in forming a body of socialist doctors' to get in touch with him.

There was an immediate response and a preliminary meeting late in September 1930, presided over by Miss Esther Rickards, MS, FRCS, quickly decided on setting up a new socialist organization. By November 2, a constitution, which J. S. Middleton then Acting Secretary of the Labour Party helped to frame, was ready to be accepted by a meeting over which Somerville Hastings, MP for Reading, presided. He had decided that it was necessary to take a more political line than that taken by the State Medical Service Association. Hastings and Brook were agreed that if any success was to be attained a Socialist Medical Association must be affiliated to and must exercise its influence through the Labour Party. The constitution of the new organization was framed in conformity with that of the Labour Party, and its three principal aims were set out as:

1. To work for a Socialized Medical Service both preventive and curative, free and open to all.
2. To secure for the people the highest possible standard of health.
3. To disseminate the principles of socialism within the medical and allied services.

It is of interest that the World Health Organization when it was established many years later declared that 'the enjoyment of the highest attainable standard of health is one of the fundamental rights of every human being'.

The founder members of the new organization spent some time discussing its name but were finally unanimous in favour of 'The Socialist Medical Association'. It began to attract attention from the day of its foundation. The time was undoubtedly ripe but it also gained notice from the names of many of its first members. They were already of such eminence as to call for attention and represented a very broad cross section of the profession. Somerville Hastings, MS, FRCS, was already one of the most trusted members of the Labour Party but he was also a senior surgeon at a London Teaching Hospital, and surgeon in charge of the Ear & Throat Department of the Middlesex Hospital. Dr Alfred Welply, who was General Secretary of the Medical Practitioners' Union and became the first Treasurer of the SMA, was of great assistance in organization. Two Trustees were elected, although as Dr Brook recalls 'there was no property to be held in trust'. But they were in a way a demonstration of the wide support the Association had. They were Dr V. H. Rutherford who had joined the Labour Party after a period as a Liberal MP and Dr Hector Munro a life long socialist, a close friend of Keir Hardie and a man of original views in politics and medicine. On the first executive committee there were Members of Parliament, Dr Alfred Salter and Dr Robert Forgan; Dr Caroline Maule, a medical graduate of the University of California; Dr A. V. R. Menon, an Indian practitioner, Dr S. W. Jeger who later became MP for South West St Pancras; Dr Oscar Tobin (later known as Watts-Tobin) who had been first Labour Mayor of Stepney; Dr Frank Bushnell, a man of great drive and originality and Dr John Powell-Evans who after thirty years was still a member of the Executive Committee.

It is a significant fact that from that moment the Socialist Medical Association was and still is continually represented in the House of Commons: and represented by men whose worth was acknowledged by all. Alfred Salter represented West Bermondsey, but he did more than represent it. He fought for it and for every one of its impoverished citizens. Charles Brook writes of him as 'the most militant pacifist and dictatorial democrat I have ever known'. He fought for a revolution but accepted every reform he could get while fighting and under his influence Bermondsey became a very changed and much more healthy borough.

Dr Frank Bushnell was a much less tolerant man who twice fought unsuccessfully to get into Parliament. He had been tuberculosis officer in Plymouth and when he retired became a member of that City's Council. He believed that a healthy nation would be possible only when the workers had realized that they were responsible both for personal and communal health and he founded 'The Plymouth Workers' Health Council' to advance that idea. In 1931 he expanded it into the Socialist Workers' National Health Council. The work he did was prodigious but unrewarded, partly because as he grew older he found it difficult to convey his ideas in simple form and was in such a hurry to get things done even his most devoted followers could not keep pace with him. The SMA found his views stimulating but tried and failed to persuade him that it was the better organization to do what he wanted, 'to further the knowledge of the Socialist application of Medicine to public health and well being and to demonstrate that the full advantage of socialized medicine can be enjoyed only in a socialist state'.

That phrase was to occur over and over again in SMA discussions and in one form or another created quite sharp divisions of opinion, usually at times when political discussions in the country as a whole had reached a point of climax. One of the first was when Sir Oswald Mosley formed his 'New Party', and drew one of his strongest supporters, Dr Robert Forgan, out of the SMA. He failed, however, to draw it out of the Labour Party toward which the major arguments for a socialized service were now to be directed. At the first meeting of the newly formed Executive Committee, held at the House of Commons in November 19, 1930, a Research Sub-Committee was formed and given the immediate task 'to devise practical measures for a Free Socialised Medical Service'.

The new young organization was nothing if not daring and the Research Sub-Committee invited various bodies to submit their views. Dr Brook reports his astonishment and satisfaction when the British Medical Association at once agreed and sent the then Chairman of the Representative body, Sir Henry Brackenbury, and the then Secretary, Dr G. E. Anderson, to give their views. Brackenbury had been a member of various committees with Somerville Hastings and this may have prompted the ready acceptance.

A month later, in December 1930, Lewis Silkin, later Minister of Town and Country Planning suggested that the SMA should prepare a 'Health Policy for London' and this was ready in time for the 1931 London County Council election. The organization had, as yet, no paid staff and Charles Brook recalls how he spent a part of Christmas Day at his home in Balham typing copies of this memorandum. It was work well done for it formed the basis of LCC policy when Labour won control in 1934. Somerville Hastings had a great influence over health policy in London and was for many years Chairman of the Public Health Committee: and in 1944 Chairman of the Council itself.

The SMA was no sooner founded than it was invited to join the International Socialist Medical Association (the first of two brief attempts to establish such a body). It met at Carlsbad in the spring of 1931 and the SMA was represented by Somerville Hastings and V. H. Rutherford. They reported a rather disappointing conference for they had not heard the thrilling propaganda for socialism they had hoped to hear but very lengthy talks on abortion and whether legal abortion should be performed by private practitioners or state doctors. Before another conference could be held many of the moving spirits were caught up in the struggle against Fascism and Dr Ewald Fabian who was then Secretary soon had to leave Berlin. But the SMA was to find itself involved in many international problems and remains committed to international cooperation, especially in health.

The main effort between 1930 and 1934 was to work out a statement of policy and to get that statement accepted by the Labour Party. This was done in two stages. In 1932 Somerville Hastings moved a resolution, which was carried, calling for the establishment of a State Medical Service. But thinking on the subject now advanced rapidly and at the 1934 conference at Southport the Labour Party Conference unanimously accepted an official document on a National Health Service which had been prepared by a special sub-committee which was largely composed of SMA members.

B

The Labour Party document *The Peoples' Health* carries the name of Somerville Hastings as author but also carries a warning that it had not at that time been accepted by the Labour Party as a whole. The SMA published *A Socialized Medical Service* and there are just enough differences between the two to show that the author met some differences of opinion in one of the organizations to which the drafts were presented. The SMA, at that time, thought the GP could look after no more than 2,500 people (the 1968 average is just under that figure) but the Labour Party thought 2,000 would be enough. It was in these documents that the definition of Health Centres manned by *Home doctors* was first clearly set out and it was here too that 'Group laboratories' first appeared. For the first time also a 'regional form' of unified health authority was advocated but the difficulties of reorganizing local government to achieve this were recognized and a form of county administration was mentioned as a possible unit.

It should be noted that the SMA document did not pass the Second Annual General Meeting in May 1932 without a great deal of argument. Dr Frank Bushnell was particularly concerned at 'reformist' tendencies for nowhere was there a clear recognition, to his mind, that both the workers in the health service and all other workers as possible patients, should share control of most parts of the service. There was a little doubt in the minds of some members as to the wisdom of going for a complete service at one time rather than extending national health insurance first and following up with the hospital service afterwards. This same argument was still to be heard in the 1942–46 period when the lines of the National Health Service were finally laid down.

It was at this same annual meeting that many people

later to become better known in politics made their first appearance. Dr Jeffrey Samuel joined and was later to replace Dr Welply as Treasurer; and his wife Dr Edith Summerskill began her long association with politics and health in the SMA and the Labour Party. She suggested that the SMA could and should attract a great deal of notice to itself and make some money which it badly needed by properly organized social events. Such an idea is always welcomed and, as always is handed back to the proposer for the necessary action. So began 'Someda', a series of dinner-dances held in conjunction with the Annual General Meetings for the next five years. They attracted not only the members but many well known political figures. Clement Attlee, Herbert Morrison, Christopher Addison, J. R. Clynes, Arthur Greenwood, Ellen Wilkinson and J. B. S. Haldane all attended. The Labour Party was recovering from its setback of 1931 and this was a period of great activity for all in the political field.

In order to broaden the appeal to members each annual meeting was planned to include a 'Popular Lecture' and some of those proved over the years to be exceedingly valuable in setting the trend of opinion. In 1934 Esther Rickards spoke on the need for a National Maternity Service and provoked such a discussion that a special meeting was held in the following November to thrash out a detailed policy. On most heads there was general agreement but Miss Rickards and Dr Summerskill took opposite views on the proportions of hospital and domiciliary midwifery a service should plan for and what qualifications those doing midwifery should hold. Dr Charles Brook says 'this started the campaign for safer motherhood in Britain and thus it can be reasonably claimed that the SMA was the organization primarily responsible not only for making the nation conscious of the needlessly high rate of maternal mortality and morbidity, but for providing the initial drive for the subsequent legislation which had such remarkable results'. Esther Rickards became a member of the LCC Health Committee (and many other bodies) while Edith Summerskill included the subject in her increasing platform appearances.

The SMA memorandum, *A National Maternity Service* was printed as a supplement to *The Socialist Doctor* which was then appearing, rather spasmodically, as funds permitted, under the editorship of Dr David Stark Murray. Dr Brook in *Making Medical History* recalls that Dr Murray had attended the inaugural meeting of the SMA (he had also attended the terminal meeting of the old SMSA) and was elected to the EC in 1931. The son of a former Scottish Labour and Cooperative MP, poet and journalist, he was soon drafting documents and when the publication of *The Socialist Doctor* was proposed was at once appointed editor. 'Owing to financial stringency very little money could be spared for this publication and, eventually, through lack of support, it slowly petered out.' But later pages will report how it was replaced by a better and more permanent journal. In the years that followed David Stark Murray became both recorder and stimulator of developments in the SMA and wrote hundreds of articles for newspapers under his own name and a number of pseudonyms. (This history is the final outcome of that work.) The propaganda, by written and spoken word, which the SMA carried out in its first fifteen years was not only intense because it was directed to one single aim but was continuous and of surprising volume.

From the moment it first met the Executive Committee of the SMA recognized that it would need a 'local' organization as well as a national body if its propaganda was to be effective. Before the end of 1930 a London and Home Counties Branch was formed with Dr Morgan Finucaine as Chairman and Dr J. Powell-Evans as Secretary. In the same year the Association acquired an Honorary Solicitor, a link which has been maintained with the legal profession ever since. The SMA was fortunate from the start in having many prominent women doctors and other health workers as members. In 1931 Dr Caroline Maule, an American physician working in London, acted as assistant Secretary. Miss Esther Rickards led most discussions in midwifery and Miss Amy Sayle on social welfare problems. As we have already noted Dr Edith Summerskill plunged into money raising activities and Dr Dorothy Arning was for a long time member of the EC. Miss Helen Keynes was always prominent in discussions of mental health.

In 1935 the SMA took a very important place in Labour Party affairs when ten of its members stood as candidates in the General Election. They were Christopher Addison, Wm Bennet, Charles Brook, Somerville Hastings, Elizabeth Jacobs, S. W. Jeger, R. A. Lyster, Alfred Salter, Sam Segal and Edith Summerskill. It was not a good year for Labour; only Dr Alfred Salter was elected. Dr Addison later became a Peer, and at the time of writing this book two of the ten, Drs Segal and Summerskill are in the House of Lords. It is also of interest that the SMA attracted many Medical Officers of Health, a group who did not normally show their own political opinion. Dr Lyster, a founder member was joined by Dr Victor Freeman (who was Chairman of the EC in 1969) and Dr Sam Leff, a great worker for socialism and for health until his premature death in 1964.

During the next two years the SMA began to feel the pressure of political events on the continent of Europe and was soon busy trying to assist refugees from Austria, Germany and Czechoslovakia. The 1933 annual conference protested against Hitler's persecution of medical workers for political and racial reasons and sent aid to victims of Nazi and Fascist persecution. At home arguments for health service developments continued and in 1936 the SMA submitted its views to the Voluntary Hospitals Commission whose Chairman was Viscount Sankey. Dr Brook records that 'Somerville Hastings dealt with the need for properly equipped and adequately staffed convalescent hospitals, Esther Rickards urged the necessity of establishing an appointments system in hospital out-patients departments, while I advocated the creation of a central bureau for arranging for the immediate admission to hospital of urgent cases and the pooling of beds for this purpose'. All these ideas were accepted and in particular the Emergency Bed Service for London was inaugurated as a result of the Commission's report.

Half way through 1936 there arose a pressing need for medical aid for the Republican forces in Spain. The SMA was soon involved in an all out effort to send people and materials but the idea of setting up a Spanish Medical Aid Committee came from Dr Brook on whose shoulders most of the work was to fall. His first approach was to Arthur Peacock who was then running the National Trade Union Club and because of his ready support that became the headquarters of all the Spanish Medical Aid activity. A very hurriedly summoned group met on the Saturday prior to August Bank Holiday and agreed unanimously to set up and work for a Spanish Medical Aid Committee. Dr Brook thought he had done enough in suggesting the committee but by unanimous request became the Honorary Secretary. The majority of the Committee were members of the SMA. Dr Christopher Addison became President, Dr H. B. Morgan, who was medical adviser to the TUC, became Chairman, and Somerville Hastings the Vice-Chairman. Among the other medical members were Harry Boyde, Michael Elyan, J. A. Gillison (LCC) P. D'Arcy Hart, Tudor Hart, S. W. Jeger, R. L. Worrall and Professor R. Marrack. Non medical members included Ellen Wilkinson, Leah Manning, Isabel Brown, Arthur Peacock and the Joint Treasurers, Viscount Churchill and Viscountess Hastings. There was of course opposition to the idea but the Albert Hall was taken for a meeting and Lord Addison presided over a crowded hall. As Chairman, Dr H. B. Morgan had a very heavy task, particularly since he was a Roman Catholic and found himself opposed by pro-Franco elements in the Church. His position as medical adviser to the TUC proved very useful in getting certain kinds of assistance. Somerville Hastings spared no effort in time or money to get the Committee moving.

With such fervour was the cause supported and so much money came in that it was decided something better could be done than simply sending supplies of medicine and dressings. This was to send a completely staffed and equipped Medical Unit and in just three weeks volunteers had been found, vehicles purchased and equipped and the unit was ready to leave. On Sunday August 23, 1936, thousands turned out to accompany and cheer the first British Medical Unit as it went from New Oxford Street to Victoria Station. There in the presence of a very large crowd, including many of London's Mayors, Arthur Greenwood and Alan Findley, then Chairman of the General Council of the TUC, despatched the Unit with valedictory speeches.

Dr Brook remained Honorary Secretary of the Spanish Medical Aid Committee until the end of 1936 when its work called for a full time Organizing Secretary. George Jeger, later MP for Winchester was appointed. This committee kept up supplies and found new volunteers until the end of the Spanish Civil War, and was then responsible for bringing to this country doctors and other medical workers who would have been in danger if they had stayed in Spain. Among them was Professor Trueta, already renowned for his surgical work, who settled in this country and became Professor at Oxford. Many lessons were drawn from the war in Spain, where SMA members were in the front line with their surgical and blood transfusion units. One of them, Dr R. S. Saxton, in the issue of *Medicine Today and Tomorrow* of March 1939 put forward the proposal, later implemented by the Government, that a civilian National Blood Transfusion Service should be set up at once 'if we are not to be at the mercy of hasty improvisations should hostilities break out'. Thirty years later that article reads like a description of what we actually do today and under the NHS the transfusion service has fully justified Dr Saxton's claim that 'when the Service has been established the fruits of our experience in Spain will enable us to make of it something of inestimable value in the practice of modern surgery'.

It was indeed the knowledge gained in Spain by its own members which led the SMA to take up and publish pamphlets on a number of war-medicine topics we will note in a following chapter. But the years 1937–39 were years of enormous effort by the SMA collectively and by individual members. It was at this time that the re-examination of policy and the elaboration of new schemes were most actively pursued and the SMA was leading medical opinion in nearly every field. It had, of course, the invaluable asset that its committees were never lopsided but always had the benefit of paramedical personnel, and many laymen with wide experience, sitting with medical men and women. It took a far wider view of problems than any purely medical group could possibly do.

At the same time it could put up teams on many topics whose names were already acceptable in public and in professional circles. General medicine was carried by such experts as Dr Horace Joules, Dr Hugh Gainsborough, Dr Richard Doll, Dr Alan Jacobs, Dr Donald Court, Dr Duncan Leys; Ophthalmology by Professor Arnold Sorsby and George Black; Chest diseases by Dr Philip Ellman, Dr B. K. Cullen, Dr Francis Jarman, and many others; Pathology by Professor J. Marrack, Dr G. Signy, Dr D. Stark Murray, Dr Harry Winner, Dr H. Voss, Dr Len Crome and so on; Psychiatry by Dr Leslie T. Hilliard, Dr Elizabeth Bunbury, Dr Brian Kirman; and general practice by practitioners from all over the country. Many were very prominent in their BMA and Medical Practitioners' Union local branches. Dentistry was well covered, and opticians were especially active.

The Second World War was to produce many portents of change but it is doubtful if the health services would ever have advanced as they were to do if the SMA had not been busy during the whole period supplying material for discussion and supplying speakers for innumerable meetings. It was something of a phenomenon not always remembered that war did not suppress but rather stimulated public desire for debate on social problems. A glance at the SMA press cuttings

book for the period shows that meetings on health and
health service questions were being held all over the
country and the SMA speakers were in continuous demand. But it was in the years 1937–39 that the policies
were elaborated that carried right through to the 1946
Health Service Bill.

THREE

1937-1942

THIS WAS A TIME OF EXPANSION in thought, in action, in total membership and in the quality of leadership so far as the Socialist Medical Association was concerned. The SMA now had many professorial figures connected with its work. Major Greenwood and J. R. Marrack were very active members and support was always forthcoming from figures like John A. Ryle, J. M. Mac-Intosh, W. Nixon. Younger men who were later to become recognized, Lipmann Kessel, Philip Wiles, Ruscoe Clarke, Lindsay Neustater, T. O. Garland, were making their progressive views known. Outside the Association there was growing recognition of the need for change in the health services and this was increased by the growing fear of war and the need for thinking out how the medical and allied professions would meet the challenge if it came. The British Medical Association was discussing and was publishing its views, the hospitals were getting together under the Nuffield Provincial Hospital Trust in ways that were new; the organization PEP was preparing a report on the health service which was to provide facts and figures for many debates, the staff at the Walton Hospital, Liverpool, were winning an award for the best plan for reorganizing our hospitals, and the SMA was preparing to launch *Medicine Today and Tomorrow*.

The SMA idea of having a journal had not been dropped, in spite of the failure to establish *The Socialist Doctor* on a permanent basis. Dr David Stark Murray had been increasing his own personal contact with newspapers and magazines and was continually writing articles on health service problems. He realized that the SMA needed a journal if its members were to be given the information they needed, that there was an element of professional journalistic skill needed which no one in the SMA possessed and that some advertising revenue is essential to running a magazine. So he proposed, and the SMA agreed, to try to establish a monthly magazine, *Medicine Today and Tomorrow*, and found the needed help from a skilled journalist, Leonard C. J. McNae, then and until his retirement in 1967, on the editorial staff of the Press Association. He was anxious to contribute something to the Labour movement and offered his unremunerated services to the new magazine. Dr Murray had close contact with *Reynolds News* and through it was able to get the assistance of Alan Hutt, recognized as a leading expert in typography, to design the journal and advise on the types to be used. Ambitious schemes for circulation were worked out, a fund was raised by SMA members and the first issue appeared in October, 1937.

Medicine Today and Tomorrow continued until the end of 1965 when its title was changed to *Socialism & Health* which the EC of the SMA thought gave a better interpretation of its purpose than the older title. Its story is embodied in its own pages. Its impact was greater than could have been calculated, its place now is as a source of information on the development of socialist thought in the field of health over nearly thirty years. Its first format, with ample illustrations, was too ambitious for an organization not able to subsidize it heavily and the advertising revenue never became adequate. War would have made its continuation on that basis exceedingly difficult; but wisdom and the advice of the new Treasurer of the SMA, Dr Leslie T.

Hilliard, reduced its size, cut it down to a quarterly but still left it of sufficient size and frequency to record new advances in medical care and to keep the SMA programme in front of an expanding audience. At the same time *Medicine Today and Tomorrow* ceased to be the official organ of the SMA which gave it editorial liberty and absolved it from publishing the more internal news of the SMA (which was issued as a separate *Bulletin*); and in the hope of developments in circulation it was handed over to a Friendly Society, Today and Tomorrow Publications Ltd. Events to be recorded in a later chapter led to all this being reversed and *Medicine Today and Tomorrow* reverted to being the official journal of the SMA with its name changed to *Socialism & Health* but continued to be edited as before.

At the start the new journal revealed how far spread was the interest in developing some form of organized health service. Articles poured in and in its first few numbers contributors included Alfred Cox, Secretary of the London Public Medical Service; Sir Daniel Hall, formerly Chief Scientific Adviser to the Ministry of Agriculture; David Forsyth, Physician to Charing Cross Hospital; Edward R. C. Walker, then Hon Secretary to the Aberdeen Branch of the British Medical Association; and Major Greenwood, Professor of Epidemiology, London University. Expert contributions were also found in fields of occupational disease, from overseas contributors like Joseph and Phyllis Gillman of Johannesburg, on medical and educational films, in books and increasingly on the threat of war.

While calling on 'medical men and women to do all that is in their power to convince both peoples and their rulers that War must be avoided at all costs', the Editor condemned the whole Fascist movement and endeavoured to alert doctors as to what was happening to the Jewish doctors of Germany, Austria and Czechoslovakia. As war drew nearer every medical aspect of modern warfare, use of gas, defence against high explosive bombs, evacuation of populations were all examined and weaknesses in Government proposals exposed.

One contributor to *Medicine Today and Tomorrow* whose writings were known over a wide circle was Dr Irwin Brown. His regular articles in *Reynolds News* and in a whole range of magazines, journals and daily newspapers were quite a feature in propaganda both for a national health service and for education in many fields of health. The present writer has to confess, with appropriate blushes that Dr Irwin Brown, and a number of other names, were pseudonyms for Dr D. Stark Murray. When variety was needed in the pages of *Medicine Today and Tomorrow* both Dr Murray and Leonard McNae attempted a variety of styles and tackled a variety of subjects. The journal appeared monthly for just one year and then as a quarterly for some years. In its third form it appeared every two months and *Socialism & Health* has continued at that frequency. It was, however, supplemented by the issue of a monthly *Bulletin* which now became the official publication of the SMA, leaving *Medicine Today and Tomorrow* available for the printing of longer statements of policy but also being free editorially to explore all new ideas on the organization of health services. It can be claimed with certainty that most of the ideas later incorporated in the NHS, and many still being discussed after twenty years of that service, first appeared in *MTT* as its readers called it.

Thus the first issue of the new series, March quarter 1939 carried *The Walton Plan*, a historic document in the growth of health service thinking. This was the

work of Dr Henry H. MacWilliam, then Medical
Superintendent of the Walton Hospital, Liverpool,
hence the name given by the Editor of *MTT* to this
plan for a National Medical Service. It was a hospital
orientated plan, but a vastly different type of hospital
from any that then existed. It was to be a district general
hospital but the words *district* and *general* took on new
meanings. Each was to have its chain of health centres
and each was to have a group of house doctors on its
staff. Team work was to be the theme and every speci-
ality was to be covered, including psychiatry (to be
served by an acute treatment unit such as was only
accepted as essential some twenty-five years later).
For each 100,000 people in areas so designed that 'the
hinterland' of cities had the same service as the centres,
there were to be 1,200 beds staffed by 84 whole time
medical officers including 33 general practitioners.
The figures in this plan would no longer be considered
adequate but at that time no better estimates were
available or had ever been accepted. The Walton Plan
strongly advocated that all doctors in a national service
should be whole time salaried employees in sharp
distinction from the views of the British Medical
Association which was still asking for a capitation fee
system for general practitioners but had moved forward quite a long way in its 1938 booklet *A General
Medical Service for the Nation.*

Meantime, the Socialist Medical Association was
moving forward and growing in membership. Dr
Charles Brook had felt it necessary in May 1935 to give
up the Honorary Secretaryship because of the growth of
his own medical practice. His place was taken by Dr
D. F. Buckle who was an Australian working in Britain.
He held the position until the approach of War forced
him to return home. It was just before Dr Brook's

resignation that two new members joined the Executive and began work for the Association which was to transform it over the next twelve years and who were to give thirty years service to it. They were Drs Leslie T. Hilliard and Elizabeth Bunbury, husband and wife, and both with strong political views which to them meant complete commitment to any task they undertook and who were by temperament and experience exceedingly able organizers. At the 1938 Annual Conference Dr Hilliard was appointed Treasurer and Dr Bunbury, Editor. Dr Bunbury during that year began the editing of the *Bulletin* of which four numbers appeared in duplicated form. The *Bulletin* was then enlarged and continued in duplicated form for 23 issues up to December 1940. That the *Bulletin* met with approval was shown by the decision of the 1939 Annual Conference that Dr Bunbury should become Propaganda Secretary. That annual conference elected to the EC three new members, Dr Mary Gilchrist who was later to do valuable work in nutrition and public health, Dr G. B. Shirlaw, whose book *Casualty* based on his two years service in Spain greatly influenced thinking on the subject of air raid casualties, and Dr G. de Swiet, a general practitioner very active politically in Kensington where he practised, and where he was later to be Mayor.

War was now imminent and the SMA took an increasing interest in the effects war would have on health. The 1939 Annual Conference passed resolutions demanding bomb proof shelters for all, pointing out the futility of much that was being proposed: and asked that hospitals should be organized as a single service to deal with all air raid casualties. There was close collaboration with many other organizations who had been alarmed by the statement of the then Minister of Health, Dr Walter Elliot, that 'possibly a quarter of a million casualties would have to be dealt with in England within three weeks of the outbreak of a war'. A joint committee was set up by the SMA, the Universities Labour Federation and the Left Book Club Medical Group, to prepare and publish *War and the Medical Services* which concerned itself not only with bombing questions but with nutrition, the effects of evacuation on children and the danger of tuberculosis in war time conditions.

During 1938/39 the SMA became increasingly involved in the question of refugees. Medical men and women were arriving daily from European countries, and the end of the Spanish Civil War brought to Britain some 250 doctors and 500 nurses who had been with the anti-Franco forces and included some who were disabled. The SMA started a campaign to assist these people and appointed Dr Mary Gilchrist and Professor J. R. Marrack to be Joint Secretaries of the Refugee Committee. War problems increased rapidly and early in 1939 a China Medical Aid Committee was formed, with Dr Mary Gilchrist acting as secretary of this also, and a great effort was made to send medical men and nurses to give much needed help in China. But most SMA members were anxious to avoid war entirely and in the name of suffering humanity to replace it as a means of settling international problems with some other system. So we find in June 1939 Dr Mary T. Day as Honorary Secretary and Professor John A. Ryle as President, asking SMA members to support the Medical Peace Committee.

But the work of the SMA was still chiefly to advocate a new form of medical care and we find it putting forward to the Labour Party Annual Conference a resolution to 'reaffirm the Party's previous decisions to make a

Socialist Medical Service part of its programme and policy'. Branches of the SMA had now been formed in South Wales, Sheffield and Birmingham. The latter owed its origin to Dr C. C. Bradsworth who had returned from two years service in Spain. The branch he formed has remained among the most active in the country. Other changes were taking place as Dr Buckle had to return to Australia and his place as Honorary Secretary was taken by Dr Brian H. Kirman. It will be recalled that the political situation at the end of 1939 was exceedingly confused and the SMA like all political organizations was divided in its attitude to the war, and especially to the position taken up by Russia.

However, *Medicine Today and Tomorrow* sought to keep the aim of the SMA firmly on its principal goal, 'a new system of medical care'. For this, it declared in December, 1939 'both the profession and the public are clamouring as to the lines along which it is suggested medicine should develop'. A committee of the SMA had been working on a document for some time which would provide 'a précis of the development of British medicine, of the most important changes taking place in other countries and of the most important schemes for the future'. This document, *Whither Medicine?* began with concepts still being argued over thirty years later. 'The family doctor,' it said, 'must always remain the most important link in the medical chain as the person whose business it is to recognize disease in its earliest form and to act as friend and adviser in all matters of health.' This he could do only if he was active in the prevention of disease and if he had 'available all hospital and specialist facilities'. Those who are still arguing about how the health service should be administered would be interested in the solution offered in *Whither Medicine?*, 'that the country should be divided into regions, which may include a number of local authorities and in which all hospitals, personnel etc, will be pooled for the common use of the whole region'.

It is doubtful if any better statement of the principles of a National Health Service was ever given than in this document: and in practice the departures from these principles proved to be minor. The writers claimed 'substantial agreement that:

1. The Service must be complete, domiciliary, institutional and specialist.
2. The patient must be freed from every economic barrier between himself and health.
3. The doctor must be given security; opportunity for advancement, for study and for leisure, and must be able to command for his patient complete medical care irrespective of his financial position.
4. The family doctor must be closely associated with the hospitals, and so far as possible be part of the same service as his consultant colleagues.
5. The hospitals and medical services generally must be regionally organized according to the density of population.
6. To ensure uniformity administration must be under the control, direct or via the local authorities, of the Minister of Health, but the doctor must be given the maximum amount of freedom in his purely clinical work.'

War now engulfed Europe and sometimes the plea for, and the advocacy of, a national health service seemed a little remote from the events of the day. Yet the membership of the SMA was growing rapidly, young doctors serving in the armed forces were developing new ideas about the kind of health services they wanted and politicians were thinking about health as one of the things they could promise 'after the war'. The next five years were to be the busiest in the existence of the Socialist Medical Association but also the most triumphant.

The Annual Conference of the SMA for 1940 was held at the end of May and among the officers a new Vice-President was appointed, Dr Horace Joules, who was to be a great source of strength for the next twenty years. As Medical Superintendent, a title he thought inadequate to describe his duties, at one of the largest and most progressive County Council Hospitals he was to give the SMA many new ideas on health service administration and above all on aspects of occupational health and air pollution. At the same meeting Dr Charles Brook, who had now become a member of the London County Council, was guest speaker with a lecture on 'Post-War Problems of the GP'. At this time no one ever accused the SMA of putting forward schemes that were not completely practical, for many of its members were not only working in the health services but actually on controlling committees. It was, for example, announced just at the time of this annual meeting that Mr Somerville Hastings and Miss Esther Rickards had again been appointed chairman and vice-chairman respectively of the Hospital and Medical Services Committee of the London County Council.

This 1940 Annual Conference was very sharply divided on the general political situation, as distinct from its unity on all matters concerned with health. The relationship of the Soviet Union to Germany, and the actions the USSR had taken, were argued over in a resolution which sought to support the Russian position and in amendments which took the view that German Fascism had to be opposed. The Editor of

Medicine Today and Tomorrow supported the latter view as he had already done in an editorial in which he quoted Litvinov as saying 'No international principle can ever justify aggression, armed intervention, the invasion of other states and the violation of international treaties.' The Annual Conference first voted in favour of the resolution, which would have meant the SMA opposing the official view of the Labour Party on a non medical matter, but later decided that this was something on which a postal ballot of all members should be held. As a result the resolution was heavily defeated.

The Summer of 1940 was busy with a great variety of events. Refugee doctors were entertained at a Garden Party at Richmond and funds for many purposes were raised. The aerial attacks on London showed that the SMA had been right in demanding a better policy for shelters and medical services and these matters were the subject of leaflets that had a wide distribution and of a well attended meeting at Conway Hall. Mr Ritchie Calder, (later Lord Ritchie Calder) strongly supported the SMA point of view on Casualty Services in the *Daily Herald*, and later in his book, *The Lesson of London*. At this time the SMA began to find support for its ideas from a very wide range of the best political and scientific brains in the country.

The concept of a socialized health service captured many imaginations and so great was the demand for ideas that *Medicine Today and Tomorrow* once again, September, 1940, summarized SMA views in a pamphlet, *Medicine Tomorrow*. This recognized that 'a completely socialized medical service will be possible only in a completely socialized community, *yet there is no reason why medicine should not be in the vanguard of the march forward*, based as it is on service and imbued with altruism and no reason why it should not be an example of the benefits to be derived from State organization'.

From the start of 1941 that march forward was to accelerate. The SMA members felt that in addition to the policy discussions in *MTT* they wanted more details of the Association's activities and it was decided that the *Bulletin* should now appear as a printed document. The Editor, Dr Elizabeth Bunbury, opened the first edition of the new series with a remark that the war was bringing fresh problems but 'courage rises with occasion'. It took some courage to start printing even four pages of printed material in war time but the SMA membership was rising rapidly and the whole political atmosphere was changing in favour of changes in the medical services, and somehow funds were found for this purpose.

The change in atmosphere was so great that in February 1941 the British Medical Association decided that it needed guidance as to the future and set up a Medical Planning Commission. The BMA sought to make this widely representative and so included three well known members of the SMA, Mr Somerville Hastings, Dr D. Stark Murray and Dr H. H. MacWilliam. All were at that time active also in the BMA, and Dr Murray was President of the Surrey Branch. Their appointment was a measure of the support the SMA had within the profession and a recognition that some changes were inevitable and that the BMA should be aware of what the Labour Party was likely to plan. *Medicine Today and Tomorrow* also claimed some credit since it had always said that 'planning should be done as a whole and should be done by the medical profession'. The Editor who was to be a member of the Commission had nothing but welcome for a body 'to study wartime developments and their effects on the country's medical services' which, while it indicated the BMA did not want to push 'planning' to its logical conclusion would still give an opportunity for others to put forward new ideas.

It is true that the Medical Planning Commission was from the start solely medical and so almost solely concerned with things as seen through doctors' eyes. *MTT* would have liked it to include 'students, the newly qualified, the young men in the Services and the EMS and GPs who were not members of the BMA'. It included, in addition to those mentioned above, Dr Haden-Guest MP, and Dr Harry Boyde who were also members but better known in other capacities, the former in Parliament, and the latter as a vocal member of the Stratford Division of the BMA. There were seven or eight other members, appointed as nominees of various bodies, who were active supporters of the idea of an organized national service of some kind. The Commission was a very large body, nearly seventy members, and was to do most of its work through sub-committees, on which the SMA members were all exceedingly active. The Editor of *MTT* expected much more from this body than was ever to appear. 'The Commission will also have to consider the cost of our medical services . . . and make a calculation as to how much we might reasonably expect to spend per head of the population.' It was suggested that the whole question of both rebuilding hospitals and rehousing people would need to be tackled and that farming policy and the use of the land would be included in a discussion of nutrition. 'A medical commission,' an article went on, 'cannot take any other view than that an optimum diet must be guaranteed by the State.' This was deliberately naïve and doomed to disappointment:

but it was surely quite realistic to hope that the Commission would in the end support or even recommend for all citizens 'a simple and easily controlled service which will preserve health and place at their ready disposal all that modern medical science offers for the treatment of disease'.

Had the Commission been allowed to go on to its own conclusion it would certainly have worked out such a scheme, and a minority report backed up by twelve to fifteen influential signatures would have stated the case for a fully socialized and salaried service. As it was it had met only a few times when it was obvious that it was proceeding very much further than its terms of reference suggested and would, whatever its conclusions, face the BMA with the alternative of accepting an advanced political view or of repudiating its own Commission. So a 'Draft Interim Report' was published in the *BMJ* of June 20, 1942 and presented to the profession at a conference, with the suggestion that the Commission might re-examine its views 'in the light of discussion and criticism'. The *British Medical Journal* recognized that there might have been at least one minority report if conclusions had been final and thought that 'divergencies can be revealed without the presentation of reservations by one or more signatories'. The SMA members had accepted that position, for the time being, and in expectation of renewed battles before the final reports appeared: but the BMA could not face up to that and the Commission never met to finalize its work. In a brief discussion at the Council of the BMA on June 10, 1942, Professor R. M. F. Picken, who was a member of the Commission, urged that the BMA must reach solid conclusions on basic principles for if, he said, 'the Association took a merely *non-possumus* attitude towards changes, then it would be in the same

position in which it had unfortunately been before, of
fighting rearguard actions against what other people
regarded as progress'. This was a prophetic utterance
which was to be true many times over in the next
twenty-five years.

Meantime the SMA had continued its work of
propaganda in public and inside the Labour Party.
Medicine Today and Tomorrow carried many articles that
clarified the question of what kind of health service
should be planned to follow the war. One pinpointed
the question of cost and was to have repercussions when
the national health service bill was finally put before Parliament. *If the Medical Services are Free, what will be the cost?*
was the first real attempt to set out the subject and reach
positive conclusions; and so well did L. T. Hilliard and
L. C. J. McNae make the calculations that they became
the basis of the financial memorandum which was presented to Parliament. By the time the first year's
actual cost of the NHS was ascertained in 1949 there
was quite an outcry at the enormous increase, as it was
forgotten that Hilliard and McNae had given their
figures at 1938–39 values which bore little relation to
the inflated values of 1948–49. It was estimated that
just before World War II England and Wales were
spending £140 million a year on a variety of health and
medical services. 'For the same expenditure', the
authors said, 'the existing medical services could be re-
organized and coordinated to provide a better average
service for the country as a whole.' Naturally they were
thinking of a salaried service and thought GPs would
average £1,000 a year but a net income as they would
'not have to provide their own secretaries, dispensers,
surgeries, cars, or instruments'. As buying of practices
would cease to be legal doctors would not need to
borrow capital and would also earn a very good

pension. The authors were ready to admit that some items of their budget might prove a little inaccurate but on the whole were satisfied that the same £140 million could be spent to far greater advantage: and an end made to the frequent remark that a national service was impossible because 'it would be too expensive'.

War problems still occupied a great deal of SMA time. At the Annual Conference of May 1941 Ritchie Calder gave the main address on 'The Effects of War on the Medical Service', foreshadowing some of the changes that could be expected. At this same meeting Dr Brian Kirman resigned and Mr Aleck Bourne was appointed Honorary Secretary in his place. Dr Bunbury reported that the *Bulletin* was not only fulfilling its primary purpose but attracting so much attention that she proposed it should be doubled in size; one part, the original *Bulletin* continuing for members only and the second to be distributed to interested laymen outside the Association. This arrangement continued until 1950 and both publications need to be consulted for details of the work that was done during those years. In spite of war the activities were constant and of great variety. We note two garden parties in 1941, at the homes of Dr D. Stark Murray in Richmond, and Dr P. A. Gover at Highgate. The first of these coincided with the entry of the USSR into the war against Hitler. The Association at once sent a telegram to Mr Maisky then Ambassador in London asking him to convey fraternal good wishes to the health workers of the Soviet Union. In a reply thanking the SMA for its good wishes Mr Maisky spoke of the need to 'strengthen and increase the cooperation between our two countries'.

Two problems on which the SMA had particular influence were those of nutrition and of tuberculosis.

Medicine Today and Tomorrow in June 1941 published a report prepared by a special sub-committee on 'The War, Tuberculosis and the Workers', which was revised and reprinted in 1942. Drawing on the figures for World War I, from Britain and from Germany, it very clearly made the point that industrial conditions caused an increase in tuberculosis and in war the increase might be disastrous. The document called for the use of mass radiography among industrial workers but also recognized that the social and financial problems had to be tackled at the same time. A deputation led by Mr Hastings put these views to Sir William Jameson, Chief Medical Officer at the Ministry of Health.

A long memorandum on the whole subject of Nutrition was sent to the Minister of Food, outlining the dangers of malnutrition but calling especially for guarantees of adequate animal proteins and supportive foods for pregnant women, children and adolescents and for all who were sick. But close attention was also paid to the needs of industrial workers: and in *MTT* Dr Jurgen Kuczynski argued that 'Better food for the workers means increased man-power'. He argued that it was not a case of guns instead of butter but of more guns out of providing butter and other foods to those in industry. He gave some very convincing figures from scientific sources in many countries.

Public propaganda was intensified during this period in a series of monthly meetings at the Conway Hall. In February, Dr D. Stark Murray spoke on 'An Approach to Socialized Medicine', in March Professor J. R. Marrack took 'Nutrition in Wartime' as his topic, and in April 'Medical Education and Research' was the subject to a symposium addressed by Professor A. St G. Huggett, Dr P. A. Gover and Mr J. H. T. Lawton.

The SMA membership was now 500 and the lay half of the *Bulletin* was proving so popular that it was renamed *Medical News and Views*. The August issue carried a long article on the medical services of the Soviet Union, the war effort of which was now creating interest in the way of living of the Russian people. Members of the SMA were now involved in schemes for medical aid and appeals went out not only for money, chiefly used by Mrs Churchill's Committee for Russian Medical Aid, but for instruments and other useful material.

The year 1942 began with further pressure on the authorities to give more attention to the nutrition of special groups. A memorandum was published at the request of the Parliamentary Labour Party Food Committee on the need for extra nourishment in illness, pregnancy and lactation. Particular attention was paid to tuberculosis, which in the first year of the war had increased instead of decreasing as it had been doing annually up to 1939. But 1942 was to be the year when the issue of a national health service, in principle, was to be settled once and for all. The BMA did not want its members to be faced with the report of its own Medical Planning Commission, which might be revolutionary and which it was intended should be presented to a BMA conference (as we have seen earlier in this chapter), in complete ignorance of the many proposals that were being made. So BMA Study Groups had been set up over the whole country and part of the literature sent to them for discussion was *Medicine Tomorrow* originally printed in the September, 1940, issue of *MTT* but now enlarged and revised.

The Association now found that industrial health questions were of increasing importance and held a conference on the subject when the speakers were Dr L. Fieldman, Dr T. O. Garland and Professor Hermann

Levy, the former German economist. In April a new
name appeared among SMA speakers when Dr Barnet
Stross spoke and later wrote on the subject of health in
the Potteries. He was Medical Adviser to the National
Society of Pottery Workers and to the North Staffordshire Miners' Federation and was to prove invaluable
to the SMA in this field. Social, historical and philo-
sophical aspects of medicine were presented to SMA
members in lectures by such authorities as Professor
J. D. Bernal, Professor Hyman Levy and Professor
Arnold Sorsby and many others. Social services were
for the first time clearly brought to the notice of members by a valuable memorandum prepared by the
Association of Socialist Social Workers, which was
virtually a sub-committee of the SMA.

Paper shortages now made it difficult to maintain all
the Association's publications. *MTT* had to be cut in
size and *Medical News and Views* became an occasional
instead of a monthly publication. The membership
was now over 900 and the Annual Conference asked the
EC to consider appointing a full time Organizing
Secretary. In July, Mrs Thora Sinclair-Loutit SRN
was appointed. As Thora Silverthorne she had gone to
Spain in the first ambulance unit and so met Dr
Sinclair-Loutit, the medical officer who commanded
that unit. Both were now active members of the SMA
and the EC considered itself fortunate to find, in war
time, so experienced an organizer. She found the SMA
now had a dozen active branches, some in unexpected
places. This was because evacuation of hospitals from
London had produced concentrations of doctors in
areas that previously had known little political activity
in the medical field, in Brighton and, notably, in
Ashford, Middlesex. Now everybody was talking
medical politics and the SMA continued to grow. By

October 1942 the membership was one thousand and
Bulletin 48 recorded the fact with a summary of SMA
history and activities. The issue of *MTT* of the same
date carried an up-to-the-minute restatement of SMA
policy *The Socialist Programme for Health*, the whole
organization standing poised for the publication of the
Report on Social Security to be known as the Beveridge
Report. That appeared at the end of November 1942
and will be a suitable starting point for our next
chapter.

FOUR

1943-1945

IT WAS QUITE EXCUSABLE for *Medicine Today and To-morrow* to give a cry of exaltation in its issue of December 1942. 'We began in the autumn of 1937', it said, 'with the seemingly insurmountable problem of converting the most conservative of all sections of the community to the idea of organizing medicine in some form which would remove the worst evils of existing medical practice; we find ourselves *now* in a world in which profession and public are completely agreed that only by the principle of cooperative practice can medicine give its full service to the world.' Two events had prompted this claim. The BMA had met to consider the Draft Interim Report of the Medical Planning Commission and had accepted 'the principle of group or cooperative practice', and by a small majority, 'that there should be provided a single medical service available to the whole community'. But as we have already said the Medical Planning Commission was fated not to complete its work and the profession lost an unexampled opportunity to lead a great reform.

The second reason for *MTT*'s pleasure was the publication of the Beveridge Report. It rejoiced in the assumption made by Sir William (later Lord) Beveridge that after the war 'a comprehensive national health service will ensure that for every citizen there is available whatever medical treatment he requires, in whatever form he requires it, domiciliary or institutional, general, specialist or consultant'. In this issue the Editor dealt exhaustively with the social security side of Beveridge, the assumption that Britain would so organize itself as 'to guarantee freedom from want and economic insecurity'. For *MTT* social security meant the acceptance of a national object 'to maintain for every citizen throughout the whole of life an economic standard by which optimum health and optimum capacity to give service to the State will be possible'. The Editor saw a parallelism between social security and health services which was still not attained twenty-five years later. 'The scheme must be national, there must be no difficulty placed between citizens in need of the payment of the full amount necessary for health, the scheme must be complete and cover every possible contingency, and it must be applicable with absolute equality to both sexes and all ages.' Freedom from want in what Beveridge himself had called 'a generous conception of need, the quintessence of social security' was to take much longer than the founding of a national health service. It was, perhaps, a pity that there was no Socialist Social Service Society to hammer home the principles Beveridge had laid down as there was in the case of the national health service. And it is a tragedy that no government had made use of the changes Beveridge thought essential, 'the separation of medical treatment from the administration of cash benefits and the setting up of a comprehensive medical service for every citizen under the supervision of the Health Department'.

Many people have spoken and written as if Beveridge invented the idea of such a service but as we have shown this was not so. Indeed the present writer had written two books on the subject, both of which summarized the political thinking of the time: and partly for that reason and partly because the author presented many new ideas on the subject, there was really only one worked out scheme in front of the public. It was the same scheme that was in front of Beveridge and it was that scheme which he accepted. It is clear that Beveridge had read SMA literature on the subject and the Draft Interim Report of the Medical Planning Commission, the thinking of which had been so influenced by its SMA members. Beveridge, therefore, neither invented nor worked out a plan: he made one of his famous assumptions, assumption B, which said in effect that he believed all the political arguments of 1941–42 must finally crystallize in a post war radically organized health service. I believe, is what he said, that in the post war era a *comprehensive* service will ensure that for *every citizen* there is available all the medical care he or she requires. He quoted at length and said he was in complete agreement with what the Medical Planning Commission had said, that it was essential to provide '(a) a system of medical service directed towards the achievement of positive health, of the prevention of disease and the relief of sickness' and to make this possible there must be '(b) available to every individual all necessary medical services, both general and specialist and both domiciliary and institutional'.

As the Editor of *Medicine Today and Tomorrow* pointed out in the issue of December 1943, Beveridge was not content to leave the question of what he meant by 'available' to others to interpret. He touched on the point a number of times that it must be provided 'without contribution condition', that it must be a service 'without an economic barrier at any point to delay recourse to it', and in another place that it must be provided 'to every citizen without exception and without remuneration limit'. Beveridge also clearly recognized that treatment of disease was not enough and that 'the restoration of the sick is a duty of the State and the sick

c

person prior to any other consideration'. Sir William, *MTT* said, emphasized over and over again that 'Rehabilitation is a vital part of social security'.

Beveridge was also fully aware that the kind of health service he was assuming would need to be based on health centres and it was therefore of particular interest that when the Government announced its acceptance of assumption B, the spokesman, Sir John Anderson spoke of 'the principles of group public practice at well equipped clinical centres which underlie most of the current thought on the future of family practice'. From his statement it appeared that ideas on health centres were being developed by the Government whose object was 'to ensure, through a public, organized and regulated service that every man, woman and child who wants it can obtain easily and readily the whole range of medical advice and attention'. Before that service was to be established, there were to be many difficulties and many changes of policy but there could no longer be anyone who doubted that a national health service was approaching rapidly.

The SMA meantime intensified its work. Medical education had been much under discussion and Professor John Ryle had addressed the Association on the need for changes in the social services and for a greater content of social teaching in the medical education curriculum. The SMA took this up at once and arranged a whole series of lectures at weekly intervals on aspects of public health which appeared to be largely omitted from the teaching of medical students. The lecturers included the President, Somerville Hastings, Dr Brian Thompson on tuberculosis, Dr Joan Malleson on venereal disease, Professor Hermann Levy on Social Insurance and Professor J. B. S. Haldane on statistics and occupational morbidity.

Both the *Bulletin* and *Medicine Today and Tomorrow*
now kept up pressure on the issues raised by the Beveridge report and a series of leaflets on the subject was
issued. *MTT* gave considerable space to the position
of dentistry in a national health service. All the
arguments which Beveridge had advanced for a complete medical service clearly applied equally to dentistry. But it was seen that there was a 'great shortage of
qualified personnel', and therefore priorities would have
to be worked out. 'Dentistry must be a vital part of a
comprehensive health service' and, the SMA dental
committee said, 'it should be available to every citizen,
with priority at the outset to those sections, particularly
the young, in whom dental care is most important'.
On the organizational side it advocated something still
not achieved twenty-five years later, that 'all dental
workers should be salaried officers of the service
working under terms and conditions of service nationally fixed; and the service should be provided through
health centres'.

The SMA's views on the health service implications of
the Beveridge Report were dealt with in leaflets, pamphlets and articles in the *Bulletin*. One of the occasional
numbers of *Medical News and Views* (No 13) set out the
whole argument and is one of the clearest statements
issued at that time: and one which establishes the
SMA's claim to having originated all the thinking on
the subject that was to find its way into legislation.
The BMA's attitude was hardening into a very nice
effort at double talk, claiming that it was in favour of
the imperative need for reform of the medical services,
especially for the working classes but going nowhere
near a comprehensive service for all. The Council of
the BMA had moved away from the position taken by
the Medical Planning Commission and while claiming

to support a nationally organized service thought that
'Assumption B should be satisfied by an extension of
National Health Insurance to include dependents and
others of *like economic status* and to cover consultant and
specialist services and laboratory and hospital facilities'.
This was at least an advance on the 1911 policies of the
BMA which at that date opposed the introduction of
NHI for workers below a certain income level. *MTT*
analysed this new view on health insurance and rejected it as being far short of what Assumption B
meant. The BMA's attitude was seen as an attempt to
protect the GP's economic position at all costs: the
principle aim was not only to protect private practice
but to see that the national health service provided
some of the means whereby private practice would
flourish. *MTT* recognized that a good trade union
must endeavour to negotiate the best possible terms for
its members but the BMA 'must not be allowed to
confuse the issue by claiming that its trade union function is an altruistic and objective attempt to solve the
problem of the health of the nation'. The SMA, on
the other hand, called for an immediate and binding
promise from the government that 'a national medical
service, freely available to all citizens, is an essential
feature of post war reconstruction and one on which an
immediate decision must be made'.

The SMA now had a membership rapidly approaching fifteen hundred and new and more recruits were
coming forward daily. A London Conference on Health
was held in February 1943 and the speakers included
Dr Joan McMichael, Sister Mary Morse and Dr Marc
Daniels who all spoke on the theme 'Health: What
needs to be done.' In March the Minister of Health
received a deputation from the SMA, which included
the President, Mr Somerville Hastings, Mr Aleck

Bourne, Dr Horace Joules, Dr D. Stark Murray, Dr L. T. Hilliard, Dr E. Bunbury, Dr Philip Inwald and Mrs Sinclair-Loutit. A memorandum setting out the SMA views was handed to the Minister. This was very largely echoed in a pamphlet *National Service for Health* issued in April 1943 by the Labour Party.

The SMA sent a copy of this pamphlet to every member and had a right to consider this publication a complete vindication of all its years of effort. The Labour Party, as we have noted, had accepted the principle of a universally available health service, on an SMA motion, in 1934. Now it was presenting to the public just what it would do if it won the first post war election and telling the war time government, the kind of scheme it should plan if it was to count on Labour Party support. This was a particularly outspoken statement. In its summary the Labour Party declared: (1) The nation needs a medical service planned as a whole; (2) It must be preventive as well as curative; and neither paid private doctoring nor National Health Insurance can 'deal adequately with the prevention of ill-health'; (3) The service must be complete and it must be open to all, *so that poverty shall be no bar to health*; (4) It must be efficient and up-to-date *providing for team work*—and only the community can achieve this by a planned disposition of hospitals, doctors, etc; (5) It must offer a *fair deal to doctor and patient* alike and only a system of *whole time, salaried and pensionable doctoring* will do. The scheme was to be nationally supervised, regionally planned and locally administered through linked divisional general hospitals and divisional health centres, with local health centres and other units getting right down to the local population. The scheme was worked out in much more detail than in SMA publications since it was aiming at early legislation and was planned to include an occupational health service. The tragedy was that even a post war Labour Government was to depart from this excellent scheme in an effort to compromise with professional opposition. The Labour Party thought that post war Britain would be in a position to afford such a service. 'The pre war expenditure of £140,000,000 sterling on treatment of the sick has been carefully analysed by the Socialist Medical Association and Dr D. Stark Murray. They estimate that if the service were planned as a State Medical Service we would get far more than we now get for £140,000,000.' But the pamphlet went away beyond this. Beveridge had given a slightly higher figure, £170,000,000 and the pamphlet went on, 'Even if the Beveridge figure were to be somewhat exceeded, the burden would still be a light one, having regard to the importance of the need and the size of the national income.' Labour had now put health among its priorities and concluded 'In the interests of the nation's health, vigour and happiness; in the interests of true economy; in the interests of the medical profession as well as the interests of the sick, the Labour Party appeals to every citizen to support this great reform—the organization of a National Service for Health.'

That Labour Party pamphlet had to be reprinted more than once. The SMA realized that no matter what majority of the people would now support a fully comprehensive health service it would be necessary to win the support and consent of a majority of all health workers. They were very poorly organized and served under a great variety of conditions and it was essential to bring them into the discussions which were always dominated by and argued over from the point of view of medical men. So the Conway Hall was taken for a Health Workers' Convention, in May 1943, and a very large number of delegates and visitors attended and most of the unions catering for health workers sent representatives. Somerville Hastings took the chair and the chief speakers were Dr Horace Joules who spoke on 'An Immediate Policy for the Health Services' and Dr D. Stark Murray who presented 'The Development of a Socialized Health Service'. This was an enthusiastic meeting which gave complete support to the policy put forward and was a clear indication of the way people's minds were working at this stage of World War II.

The growth of the SMA now presented its officers with organizational problems. It was decided to drop the idea of an Honorary Secretary and appoint instead a professional General Secretary. As a result Mr Aleck Bourne ceased to be Honorary Secretary and was elected as Vice President (the others were Dr Charles Brook, Professor J. R. Marrack and Dr D. Stark Murray). The Executive now became a Council and a Working Committee was appointed to control the business as apart from the policy affairs of the Association. A Drafting Committee, a Propaganda Committee and a Scientific Committee were appointed. The idea of a Council dealing with policy and an Executive dealing with administration matters became fixed. War time imposed many difficulties, one being that the Association could never get enough paper for its purposes. The *Bulletin* was reduced to a single sheet. Leaflets were possible, however, and some had a very large circulation among the many organizations supporting the Association's work. The Association clearly saw that it had to influence the medical profession as much as possible but it also had to make the public so convinced of the need for a national health service that nothing would be allowed to stand in its way.

The SMA also spent time on new ideas on the relationship between public and professions on administrative bodies. Opponents of a national health service have always used baseless arguments about the evils of socialism and this period saw an intensification of these attacks. The editor of *MTT* repeatedly tried to clarify the issues. 'We have repeatedly stressed that the terms and conditions of employment of the doctors and of all other health workers are of vital importance. They must be generous and simple and must provide for *complete clinical freedom* as well as for scientific advice and, in some matters, scientific control.' However, the democratic principle must be paramount and it was for 'the 45,000,000 people of this country for whom a complete health service is vitally necessary, to decide on the general structure of that service'. Since the public would 'have nothing to do with an extension of National Health Insurance' something quite new was needed.

This was indicated in a new exploration of the *Administration of the Health Services* which was presented to the Ministry of Health. The first point made was that a comprehensive service must be conceived as one whole and its administration must be based on this concept. 'It must function as an agreed partnership between the people and the medical profession.' That administration must be designed to enable rapid decisions, to cover town and country, and to control the quality of care given. Since Health Centres would be an essential feature of the service and family doctors would be working as a team with the cooperation of consultants at the centres, in hospital and in the home, only a full time salaried service would be suitable and that would make administration more simple and more flexible. The SMA also brought forward a point in democratic control which until the National Health Service had never been conceded, that a doctor, and by inference any health worker, 'can sit on the authority responsible for the service in which he is employed'.

It is of interest, nearly twenty-five years later to look back at this very detailed structure, for it would have avoided many errors if it had been accepted. It was assumed that Parliament would continue to have over-all responsibility for the service and that the Minister of Health would 'prepare a plan for the whole country', and that he would be advised by departmental com-mittees. The machinery would be national, regional and local, but at that time it was thought that the regional body would be appointed from people elected to a Regional Council which would have all the local government duties of regional councils. The local units were to be much more executive bodies composed of whole time medical and other officers: and any lay committee was to be of a 'watch dog' type. This docu-ment precipitated discussion all over the country and led to the development of many new ideas. Health Centres became the subject of meetings in many places and already some proposals were coming forward for 'pilot' schemes.

The SMA began 1944 with over two thousand members. There were 29 branches and groups, all engaged on active work. The Belfast branch produced its own pamphlet *Health in Belfast* which set the ball rolling on the form of an organized service for Northern Ireland. Birmingham called a conference on Health Centres and had a very large audience. In the London borough of Wandsworth the SMA branch joined mem-bers of the Trade Council to work out in great detail a plan for a health service to cover the whole borough. Some members joining the SMA expressed a need for more information on socialism as a political philosophy and in London a series of classes were held. Every member was sent a copy of *Why I am a Socialist* by John Strachey, accompanied by notes prepared by the Drafting Committee. These speaker's notes proved very useful to the increasing number of members addressing Trade Unions and other bodies. Literature was in great demand, the Electrical Trades Union, for example, sending out to its branches 500 copies of *The Socialist Programme for Health*. Trade Unions also took in large numbers *New Weapons Against Tuberculosis*, a pamphlet prepared jointly with the Labour Research Department.

In February of 1944 the fight for health took a new turn with the issue by the Minister of Health, Mr Willink, of the Government's White Paper, *A National Health Service*. This was less than had been hoped for and was to be weakened when Willink yielded to BMA demands, but it was enough to make *MTT* say 'On its basic principles the White Paper is sound.' It reminded its readers of its first editorial in 1937 when it said, 'Health is the right of every citizen, it is not a commodity to be bought by those who can afford to buy it and to be denied to those who cannot.' It therefore welcomed the Government's declaration that its policy was 'to divorce the care of health from questions of personal means or other factors irrelevant to it; to provide the service free of charge and to encourage a new attitude to health—the easier obtaining of advice early, the promotion of good health rather than only the treatment of bad . . . to provide therefore for all who want it, a comprehensive service, covering every branch of medical and allied activity'. It will be seen that though sound basic principles appear to be enunciated the language tends to be the language of compromise and the SMA called for everyone interested in a truly socialist solution to keep up pressure on the Government.

In the first debate in the House of Commons this position was made clear by the speeches of three SMA members, Dr Haden-Guest, Dr Edith Summerskill and Dr H. B. Morgan. They attacked the White Paper for its failure to accept a unified service, for leaving the small voluntary hospital almost untouched and for its proposals to maintain private practice and subsidize it inside the health service. Later, Aneurin Bevan was to make two of these errors although on private practice he tightened up the rules so that it was not to be so much something 'which in other places would be called graft, racketeering or black market'. It is true that the White Paper recognized the danger for it warned that the service must not give 'anyone reason to believe that he can obtain more skilled treatment by obtaining it privately than by seeking it within the new service'. In the end this was the point, disguised by many spurious arguments, that was to be the reason for the BMA's opposition to the White Paper and to later proposals, that a whole time salaried service of highest quality would mean the end of private practice and must therefore be fought to the end.

The second half of 1944 was full of the battle for salaried health service. The BMA arranged for a referendum of the medical profession on many different aspects of health service proposals. Only 50 per cent of the profession answered the questionary sent out and *MTT* warned that it must not be assumed that the others would have voted the same way. On the contrary 'we can safely assume', said the Editor, 'that nearly all the remaining 50 per cent agreed with and accepted the certainty of the Government scheme'; and did so to such an extent that they did not consider

it worth while answering questions which were loaded
to discover objections rather than agreements. Thus
74 per cent of consultants replied while only 29 per
cent of those employed by local authorities did so.
But when the figures were analysed, 60 per cent of
those voting (and 73 per cent of those in the services)
were in favour of a general practitioner service for all,
69 per cent in favour of a complete hospital and consultant service free to those using it and 83 per cent of
doctors in the armed forces wanted to come back from
the war to a health centre. It was even more significant
that a poll among medical students revealed that 89
per cent were in favour of Health Centres. And it was
quite astonishing that doctors did not expect very high
incomes, for 50 per cent of those replying expected
whole time salaries, with pension rights, would fall in
the range of £1,000–£1,500 per annum.

Had the Minister of Health been a socialist he would
have had at this point a mandate from the profession
to go right ahead. But he decided to give time for the
BMA to manipulate its forces and to negotiate behind
closed doors. The BMA questionary had been analysed
in age groups and it was very clear that the elderly and
more wealthy members of the profession were still
against anything that approached a national health
service. It was they, and not the young men who were
abroad with the armed forces, who formed the negotiating body; and no other group of health workers were
even asked to express their views. The SMA issued and
distributed very large numbers of leaflets, the first
A National Health Service: The White Paper explained
giving reasons why every citizen should back the White
Paper in its original form because it said that 'if people
are to have a right to look to a public service for all
their medical needs it must be somebody's duty to see

that they do not look in vain'. This leaflet recognized that a war time Government was a coalition and was likely to look for a compromise settlement to any disputes but, nevertheless, the White Paper would be a step forward. A second leaflet, *Your Health Service in Danger* was written because of the grave danger 'that pressure by those interested in keeping things as they are will force the Government to weaken its proposals and lose the opportunity to provide the people with the finest health service in the world'. The third leaflet, *Health Service or 'Panel'* was a direct attack on the BMA's attempt to restrict any changes to an extension of the existing National Health Insurance system by first giving hospital care to those already insured and then bringing in the poorer groups of women and children. The position was acute because the BMA and the Minister of Health had now drawn up a second document which in effect destroyed all that the White Paper had prepared.

It was now the beginning of 1945 and the SMA called a National Conference in London at which the attendance showed both the interest now felt in the subject of health throughout the country and how strong the influence of the SMA had become. An audience of 510 included representatives of 159 Labour Party branches, 98 Trade Union delegates and 57 from various cooperative organizations. Mr Somerville Hastings took the chair and began the meeting with letters and messages of support from leaders of the whole working class movement, including Miss Ellen Wilkinson, the Chairman of the Labour Party; Mr G. A. Isaacs, Chairman of the TUC; Mr Jack Bailey, Secretary of the Cooperative Party; and Mr Harry Pollitt, Secretary of the Communist Party. In his opening remarks Mr Hastings spoke of the White

Paper as 'preparing a good, though not a perfect, health service', and called on the Labour movement to make it clear that 'the people wanted a coordinated and complete service'. The principle speakers were Mr Fred Messer MP and Dr D. Stark Murray who presented to the audience a resolution which in effect was a preview of what the Labour Party Conference was to decide a few months later, and a Labour Government to put into force within three years.

The SMA at this time intensified its work in many fields. The end of the war still seemed a long way ahead and London and the south of England were suffering from Germany's aerial bombs. But meetings were held on every aspect of medical care. Dr Harold Baline, one of Britain's recognized experts spoke on Rehabilitation to a meeting jointly organized with the Labour Research Department; Professor J. M. Mackintosh took the Chair at an important meeting on 'Health Problems of British India', with Professor J. A. Ryle as the chief speaker. The Birmingham Branch held thirteen public meetings during 1944, with many prominent speakers. The Policy Committee pressed on with statements on many subjects, *Mother and Child* being one of the most important statements on Maternity and Child Welfare subjects ever published (*MTT*, June 1945). All of this was part of the growing desire of the British people for change and advance and the sudden announcement of a General Election offered the chance of cataclysmic changes by ordinary parliamentary methods: and the British nation grasped the opportunity and returned a Government 'for the purpose', as *MTT* put it, 'of so organizing our industries, our social services and our international relationships that Britain jumps to the front and leads all peoples to a better way of life'.

But this was presaged by the Labour Party Conference in that year when the Socialist Medical Association had the privilege of setting out Labour's policy on health in considerable details. Dr D. Stark Murray, now Vice President of the Association, moved a lengthy resolution which was accepted by unanimous acclamation, Dr Edith Summerskill, an SMA member, having the pleasure of announcing the support of the National Executive. The resolution was framed in the light of what was known of Willink's proposal to meet all objections of the BMA and other professional bodies. Conference would have none of this and declared 'that no scheme is acceptable which does not:

(a) give to local Authorities control over municipal hospitals and medical services on statutory Health Councils and Committees;

(b) accept full accountability for expenditure from public funds;

(c) end the National Health Insurance "Panel" system with its one standard of service for the poor and another for the rich, and ensure that distribution of doctors is determined by the needs of the population;

(d) give Local Authorities power of initiation and control of Health Centres;

(e) abolish the buying and selling of practices paid for by public funds;

(f) provide for the training of doctors, nurses and other health workers by using the municipal hospitals and by making medical education free to all suitable candidates irrespective of sex;

(g) include the National Health Service as part of the Comprehensive Social Security plan.'

It will be noted that at this time the SMA and the Labour Party were both thinking of the health service being controlled by some form of Local Government Authority. This resolution left the point deliberately vague for the Labour Party pamphlet already discussed had said that the health service administration would need to follow whatever changes were made in Local Government. It recommended that for Local Government 'the country should be divided into Regions, each having a Regional Authority, democratically elected'. For health purposes the Labour Party also recommended that each of these Regional Authorities should appoint a 'Health Committee for its region'. This Health Committee with appropriate sub-committees was to be responsible for the whole of the health services of its area and was to provide these on a plan which was broadly set out as Divisional Hospitals associated with Divisional Health Centres and Local Health Centres.

It will be seen that this was to be a two tier administration for the only other controlling body was to be a greatly strengthened and streamlined Ministry of Health. 'The powers of the Ministry will need revision . . . on the one hand to cover all Health Services including . . . School Medical Services and the health service in factories. On the other hand the Ministry of Health should be relieved of responsibility for services which affect health only indirectly and which involve large scale organization . . . for example housing.' In a brief discussion of what even thirty years later was still to be a debated point, the Labour Party said that the only possible central authority that could control the health service was the Ministry of Health for 'no other authority has the Ministry's accumulated knowledge of national health conditions; nor could any organization less nationwide in scope be held responsible to Parliament'. This was a direct rejection of the view put forward by some doctors that the health service should be 'taken out of politics'. The Labour Party was emphatic that 'in a matter which so vitally concerns the whole nation, it is Parliament, representing the whole nation, which must have ultimate control'. The Minister of Health, it was concluded must 'continue to be responsible to Parliament'. Health was thus seen to be the concern of the people themselves and the decisions as to how it was to operate, how staff and patients alike were to be safeguarded, how much money was to be spent on it were clearly to be political decisions. 'The Conference calls upon the Government to implement by legislation nothing less than the proposals of the White Paper as a basis of a comprehensive health service.'

The Labour Party by adopting the above resolution had thus cleared away any misconception that it was bound by the compromises Willink had negotiated with the medical profession with complete disregard for the figures obtained in the BMA's own questionary. That conference was reported in the June issue of *Medicine Today and Tomorrow* in which the Editor wrote, 'The position facing the country is that if a Tory Government is returned to power the health service proposals will be dropped' or if not dropped, modified in favour of the doctors. The election gave everyone a chance to understand that 'only the return to power of a Socialist government can give the people what they so much desire, a complete service staffed by whole time salaried officers, able to give the very best possible service; a service of which the scope, quantity and quality is determined by the people themselves, advised by doctors who are free from all the restrictions which the present economic basis of medicine places upon them'.

By the next, September, issue the Editor (who had unsuccessfully fought Richmond, Surrey in the general election) was able to claim for his journal and the SMA a triumph probably unparalleled in political history. The first post war King's Speech had told the new Parliament that in its first session 'they will be asked to approve measures to provide a comprehensive scheme of insurance against industrial injuries, to extend and improve the existing scheme of social insurance and to establish a national health service'. It was true that many battles would still have to be fought but among the 393 Labour MPs, all pledged to a national health service, there were 12 members of the SMA, 'willing and able to help the Minister of Health work out the more intricate details' of the necessary legislation.

The twelve MPs were Mr Somerville Hastings, MS, FRCS (Barking), President of the SMA who had already, for ten years been Chairman of the London Hospitals and Medical Service Committee which had been making great efforts to convert the old poor law institutions into municipal hospitals; Dr L. Haden-Guest, MC (North Islington) who had already been an MP for 12 years; Dr Edith Summerskill (West Fulham), Parliamentary Secretary to the Ministry of Food; Dr H. B. Morgan (Rochdale) medical advisor to the TUC; Dr S. W. Jeger (South East St Pancras), an LCC member since 1931; Dr Stephen J. L. Taylor (Barnet) author and formerly assistant editor of *The Lancet*; Dr L. Comyns (Silvertown) who had a staggering victory in the election, both opponents losing their deposits; Dr Barnet Stross (Hanley) medical adviser to trade unions in Staffordshire; Dr Samuel Segal

(Preston) who had a long history of political work and a notable war time record; Mr Richard Clitherow (Edge Hill, Liverpool) who had taken up medical studies after a very varied career ranging from the Canadian 'Mounties' to retail pharmacy; Captain John Baird (Wolverhampton East) son of a Scottish coal miner, practising as a dentist in Birmingham; Captain Will Griffiths (Moss Side, Manchester) a consulting ophthalmic optician who had a very distinguished war record. Mr Clitherow died soon after completing his medical studies and five others have since died. But all saw the National Health Service Act on to the Statute Book; and three are now serving in the House of Lords as life peers: Lady Summerskill and Lords Taylor and Segal. Somerville Hastings now had a strong team inside the House of Commons, all people of wide experience and able to maintain the arguments for a comprehensive service in the face of all opposition.

Outside Parliament the SMA kept up its educational propaganda. A leaflet, issued as soon as Labour was in office, called *The Health Worker and the New Britain* was directed primarily at those groups of health workers who had hitherto not been included to any extent in the discussions about their own future. The second, *Your New Health Service* was a summary of the proposals Aneurin Bevan had put before Parliament and a call to all citizens to remember, and to act upon the slogan, 'The Health of the people must be the concern of the people'. It was felt that the people would welcome all the information the SMA could give and so it was decided to prepare material for a 'Health Services Week'. This was to be in February 1946, the year of the Health Service as far as Parliament was concerned. The year 1945 had been one of climax so far as the preparatory work was concerned; now the Association had to play its part in getting the National Health Services Bill passed by both Commons and Lords. *Bulletin* 74, November–December 1945, called on every member to work as they had never worked before at this moment of 'transition from theory to practice'.

FIVE

1946–1950

THIS MOMENTOUS PERIOD opened with the preparation and staging of Health Services Week, a most ambitious project. An exhibition mounted on portable screens (which later went to many parts of the country) was backed up by fourteen lectures which had in all over two thousand five hundred in their audiences. The Exhibition was both historical and political, giving all the arguments for a national health service and was very well received by spectators and by the Press. Both at the London showing and later in provincial towns a very large quantity of SMA literature was sold. The Bill to establish the National Health Service was already published and people were clamouring for all the literature on the subject they could get.

The National Health Service Bill, the Editor of *MTT* said, falls short of the policy which that journal 'has persistently advocated, but we do not hesitate to welcome it as a great advance in the liberation of man from the bonds of economic slavery and ill health which were the lot of 90 per cent of the people of this country under the capitalist system'. The SMA hailed the main points of the Bill as a triumph for all their efforts, 'complete hospital care in a single national hospital service! Health Centres a principal objective of the scheme! A complete system of health care by a single route, a one hundred per cent service for one hundred per cent of the people!'

There were, of course, important defects which the SMA was determined to remove but which were points on which Aneurin Bevan needlessly gave in to the BMA in order to weaken their general resistance to a one hundred per cent service. It was unfortunate, *MTT* put it, that 'the Minister has not accepted the two very important principles that the service should be run by a single elected regional authority and that all officers, including general practitioners, serving with it, should be whole time salaried officers'. It was conceded by the SMA that the first point was difficult to achieve in the absence of complete reform of local government, but if a new regional authority was being set up it should control all services and not only hospitals. It was, of course, an enormous step forward, and probably Bevan's greatest decision on a disputed point, that all the hospitals were amalgamated in one system and the administrative problems were quite big enough to keep a hospital authority busy. But in the atmosphere of 1946 when people were ready for great new moves it was strange that Bevan did not see and did not grasp the opportunity to make a complete break with the past. *MTT* rightly saw the local executive councils as purely and simply a sop to the BMA.

Of course Bevan came up against the BMA very violently on this question of the authority which was to run the service. It had long been a cardinal point with doctors, especially GPs that they would not join a service administered by existing local authorities, many of which they considered 'are too small or too poor or both, to administer such services efficiently'. There was a deep seated prejudice against 'the Town Hall' which was not removed by repeated statements by Bevan and others that doctors would have complete clinical freedom whatever the administration. A new type of authority was, therefore desirable and had Bevan been able to persuade his Cabinet colleagues that such a

body could be set up for health in advance of the reform of local government, destined to be incomplete
twenty-five years later, he might have avoided the tripartite administration which was finally agreed on.
His own personal view was quite clear, as given later
in his book *In Place of Fear*, that the Minister of Health
should not have the responsibility of appointing administrative committees. 'Election,' he said, 'is a better
principle than selection' for no Minister 'can feel
satisfied that he is making the right selection over so
wide a field'. He knew that the Medical Planning
Commission had made two suggestions on this, one
very similar to the Labour Party's Health Committees
of elected Regional Authorities and a second in the
form of an appointed Regional Council drawing on
nominees of the local authorities, of the Minister and
of the medical profession. Bevan assured the BMA that
by revised units of local government he was speaking
entirely of new bodies which 'would not be local government units in any proper sense of the term'. However
in the end he was compelled to accept that 'no electoral
constituency corresponds with the functional requirements of the Service': and once the tripartite arrangements had been worked out defended them against
attacks by members of the SMA who still fought for a
unified service. So far as the medical profession was
concerned the tripartite division with a guarantee of
doctors having a place on every committee was seen as
some kind of victory and BMA opposition turned to
points concerned with 'terms and conditions of service'. Bevan enjoyed this part of the battle and was
often amused by the public utterances at BMA meetings which contrasted with what was said in committee. 'My trade union experience,' he records 'had
taught me to distinguish between the atmosphere of the

mass demonstration and the quite different mood of the negotiating table.' It is worth quoting Bevan's own summary of the relationship that should exist between the medical profession and the community. 'There is no alternative to self government by the medical profession in all matters affecting the content of its academic life, although there is every justification in lay cooperation in the economy in which it is carried out. The distinction between the two is real. It is for the community to provide the apparatus of medicine for the doctor. It is for him to use it freely in accordance with the standards of his profession and the requirements of his oath.' The SMA had understood this from the start and so their arguments with Bevan were always clearly on the subject of how best to provide the best 'apparatus of medicine'.

In the arguments about local government one point from the Labour Party's 1943 pamphlet was not challenged by the BMA, that Health Centres would be built by the local authorities. To some this appeared to give the local authorities some degree of control over general practice; in the long run it was to prove a great mistake, rectified in the Scottish NHS Act, which put the duty of building Health Centres on the Secretary for State, because reactionary County Councils joined with reactionary doctors to make the building of any Health Centres virtually impossible. It was not until after 1965 that progress was to be made in this field.

The greatest misjudgment of 1946 was the decision not to establish a whole time salaried service. The country was ready for that sort of change and had imagined Bevan had been made Minister of Health just because he was strong enough to carry through such a reform. The medical profession was sharply divided on the point and when £66,000,000 was offered as compensation for the abolition of the buying and selling of practices, the point that medicine was being taken out of the market place could have been carried to its logical conclusions. Without this, as *MTT* said, 'The new service does not appear to make sufficiently complete the break from the inefficient, disease-treatment, private enterprise system of the past and does not clearly lay down the lines on which health advice, education, promotion and preservation are to be the rule.'

The BMA opposed the national health service on many different points and the Negotiating Committee which had in it also members from other medical organizations set out as a series of 'fundamental principles' which they declared must be fulfilled in any legislation. The SMA *Bulletin* 75, January 26, 1946 declared that these had been composed entirely from the point of view of the doctors and not, as the principles laid down by SMA were, from the basis of the needs of the people. As it turned out Bevan ignored these claims in setting out his ideas and never tried to prove that he had met them but rather left the profession to quietly drop them and proceed to discussions on practical points along lines which he, the Minister, wanted settled.

The 1946 Annual Conference of the SMA spent a considerable time discussing not only the health service bill but also its own position in the belief that 'the consistent work of the Association in its sixteen years of life has contributed in no small measure to the changes in public and professional opinion', which made such a bill possible. For some years the Association had tried to run its work with a salaried General Secretary but it was felt that it was really necessary to have an Honorary

Secretary of professional and preferably medical stand-
ing. Dr Elizabeth Bunbury who had been giving an
increasing amount of time to the office work of the
Association was appointed and began five years of in-
creasingly useful work. All the newly elected MPs who
were members of the SMA were appointed Honorary
Vice Presidents. The Standing Committee (C.) of the
House of Commons just appointed to consider the
NHS Bill contained eight of these Honorary Vice
Presidents among its members.

The main debate at this Annual Conference was on a
lengthy resolution, moved by Dr Hugh Gainsborough,
and seconded by Dr Richard Doll, welcoming the NHS
Bill, accepting as a temporary provision the tripartite
administration and asking that the Bill should permit
all GPs who wished to be paid by salary to have that
right and urging that an occupational medical service
should be added to the Bill. When these points had
been carried unanimously Dr D. Stark Murray moved a
resolution, also carried without dissent, indicating that
the SMA now had two main tasks, first 'to assist the
National Health Service Bill through its legislative
stages as rapidly as possible'. The Association would
then have an educative function, 'explaining the advantages of the new Service to the public and more
particularly to our professional colleagues'.

This work became very intense around the time between the first reading and the Royal Assent to the Bill
and had two main features. On the one hand the Policy
Committee was in continuous session for the whole of
that time: and during the period when the Bill was
being considered by Standing Committee (C) the Policy
Committee met every evening and continuously put
forward new ideas and new arguments to the SMA
members of the Standing Committee. They also took

up many points with the Minister both by meeting him and by setting out questions to him. That Aneurin Bevan looked upon this exchange as important is shown by the speed with which he replied and the detailed examination of the arguments which he made. Asked about the way in which Regional Hospital Boards would work and the degree to which they would be under Ministerial control he replied: 'I want both the Boards of Governors (of teaching hospitals) and Regional Boards to be as free and flexible in administration as possible. But *both* will be working within a *planned service* settled for the region by *me* and will, and will be always, subject—as may be needed—to my directions.' To SMA objections to private pay beds he replied: 'My object in providing pay beds will be (a) to prevent encouraging a rival "nursing-home" service and (b) to attach to *my hospitals* all the leaders of the profession . . . subject to primary needs of the public service, of course.' It was during these discussions that the SMA established, much to the annoyance of part time teaching hospital consultants, that whole time doctors could be members of any board or committee, including the one under the direction of which they worked. Indeed the principle was established for all health workers but very few ever were appointed even by Bevan.

The second intensification of SMA work was in the country where the SMA's 'Battle for Health' Exhibition was in great demand not only by SMA branches but by constituency Labour Parties, Cooperative Political Committees and local Fabian Societies. Seldom was the Exhibition shown on its own, usually it was accompanied by a series of lectures and some of the officers of the SMA visited many parts of the country to address meetings. There were many requests for 'debates' but the BMA was exceedingly reluctant to put up speakers as their case was really too weak to be exposed in public. SMA speakers continually reported back to the Policy Committee on the points that came up in questions and these were dealt with if necessary by official questions and answers in Parliament. One point had to be added to the Exhibition, a description of the proposed administration, and Dr L. T. Hilliard prepared a diagram which set this out very clearly. It was reprinted many times.

For the whole of the second half of 1946 the SMA had to maintain a very steady barrage of argument against the British Medical Association which went on fighting against the National Health Service Bill. First it would not negotiate at all with the Minister of Health: then it would agree to discussions on topics it wanted to discuss but not those which had to be discussed in order to get the new service off to a flying start. When the 'negotiations' came to an end Aneurin Bevan took the unprecedented step of sending an explanatory letter to every doctor but that was not the end of the battle. The BMA kept up its theoretical objections all through 1947 and its threat of 'strike action' up to the end. But the Minister was not to be deflected and he began appointing people to Regional Hospital Boards and other committees and the BMA made sure it had its representatives on all of them. The Editor of *MTT* who was himself serving on a Regional Hospital Board wrote that 'where members of the BMA are serving on these Boards the observer is struck with the very big difference between the attitude shown and that adopted at the BMA representative meeting'. The story of how the BMA fought against the service and how the Tory Party voted against it in the House of Commons are part of the story of how the National Health Service

Act was finally passed; here we are concerned with the work of the SMA which was only in part concerned with that struggle. The SMA knew that this was an Act setting up a service which would start, not be completed, on the appointed day and that in preparing for a second Labour Government, plans 'must include the next stages in the perfection of our health and social services'.

The Council of the SMA therefore concluded 1946 with a whole day discussing a statement put forward by one of its Vice Presidents, Dr D. Stark Murray. Members did not agree with his assessment in every detail or in every emphasis but the statement was finally accepted as SMA policy for the following years. What had been achieved in the National Health Service Act was accepted as a great step forward but the SMA now had to concern itself with what had *not* been achieved. It was quite a formidable list:

(1) A unified service: the tripartite administration was certain to produce variations and gaps.

(2) No occupational Health Service.

(3) Private practice was inside instead of outside the national health service.

(4) Although the Labour Party had accepted the basic need for a whole time salaried service, the Minister of Health had not.

(5) No clear decision had been reached on the provision of staff committees which would include every grade of worker, technical, clerical and medical.

(6) No clear decision had been made about the composition of Hospital Management Committees nor about the function of part time consultants on them.

(7) No statement had been made on the need for a district general hospital to serve all sick; voluntary and municipal hospitals must be equal partners.

Many of these points could be considered only by experts but the SMA was the only organization which realized and advocated the active participation of the sick, as citizens. 'Only a lively public interest will lead to the continuous improvement of the National Health Service.' But the public had to be educated and the Policy Committee continued its work of examining the regulations which the Minister of Health was now producing and which would be the real controlling factors in the development of the service. By the end of January 1947, the BMA had agreed to enter into discussions with the Minister, the BMA thus extricating 'itself from an indefensible position and, perhaps, hoping to fight another day on strategically better ground'. In effect, however, once discussions had started they were almost bound to lead to the profession, as a whole, coming into the service for the machine had started to move and the BMA could not stop it.

At this point both the SMA and the Minister of Health thought it was opportune to come together on a more convivial note than the committee room afforded and a less formal occasion than meeting the Minister surrounded by his officers. So a dinner was arranged at which Mr Bevan was to be the guest of the evening. An enthusiastic gathering of nearly 300 listened to Mr Somerville Hastings move the toast of 'The Appointed Day' and reminded the Minister of Health that this was a moment of triumph both for the SMA and for him. Mr Bevan replied in a speech which showed full appreciation of how much he and the new National Health Service owed to the SMA and its President. Following a witty and informative speech Dr Horace Joules proposed a toast to 'The SMA members in Parliament' which was replied to by one of the new MPs Dr (later Lord) Stephen Taylor. To complete the evening Dr Charles Brook spoke of the 'SMA, 1930–1947' and Dr D. Stark Murray combined optimism and a warning in 'The SMA and the Future'.

So, as we have said, the SMA continued its educational work. Over 70,000 copies of a leaflet *Your New Health Service* were distributed and 40,000 copies of a leaflet produced by the Brighton Branch, *The People's Health: Private Profit or Public Service* were circulated. From the policy point of view the most important subject was seen to be Health Centres. In a resolution to the Labour Party it was recognized that with the need for greater house building and a start to hospital building, Health Centres could not be built in every community but the use of temporary buildings was urged and in particular 'the inclusion of plans and sites for Health Centres in all new towns and new building sites, and the building of comprehensive experimental Health Centres in several large areas of population'. There was relatively little information available as to how Health Centres would work since none built to the SMA plan existed and so the Policy Committee prepared a statement on the whole subject. 'At or through the Health centre,' it began, 'the patient will be able to secure all forms of medical care he may need, and the general practitioner will have easy access to specialist opinion and to pathological and other aids to diagnosis.'

This document, published in *Bulletin* 87, May 1947 and reissued as a pamphlet, marks the difference in attitude between the SMA and the BMA (the difference in ideas was equally marked). The BMA was fighting a rearguard battle, putting up sterile argument in favour of the *status quo* and of private practice; the SMA was thinking primarily of the patient and working out how a better service in the continually changing and expanding post war world of medical science could operate. The sub-committee which finalized this document was typical of the SMA (and again in sharp contrast to the purely medical committees set up by the BMA and other medical bodies) in that it had members representing most of the groups of health workers who might be expected to work in a Health Centre. Dr W. W. Fox, a north London GP was chairman, and three other GPs, Dr P. Inwald, Dr J. Powell-Evans and the SMA founder Dr Charles Brook were members; as were Mrs Iris Brook, SRN, Miss M. Cornelius, MPS, Miss I. Forstner, PSW, Mr L. Elmer, LDS and Mr S. R. Marcus, FBOA, representing nursing, pharmacy, psychiatric social work, dentistry and optical service respectively.

These and other health workers were seen by the SMA as vital to the success of the health service and so two issues of *Medicine Today and Tomorrow* were given over to articles by members of various professional organizations and a plea was 'made that they should work out a common policy for joint negotiations'. The March 1947 issue included as part of this series an article by Dr (now Lord) Charles Hill describing the British Medical Association and advancing some exceedingly specious arguments why it was not a trade union and could not be converted into one because the 'objects of a trade union include the "regulation of the relations between workmen and masters", and doctors were neither workmen nor masters'. But in a remark typical of the writer he went on, 'However, the BMA's purely voluntary status has not noticeably cramped its style in safeguarding the interests of the profession.' At that precise moment negotiations were going on to make all doctors in the health service except GPs salaried servants of the new health service; and by the acceptance of a departure from a pure capitation fee for GPs began the process, slow but inevitable, toward the day when even GPs would accept a salary as their method of payment.

In the same issue Dr Gordon Ward set out the policy of the genuine Trade Union of the medical profession, The Medical Practitioners Union, of which the policy was 'to press strongly for improvement in the working conditions of general practitioners in all circumstances'. The MPU considered that 'the NHS Act should be accepted as it stands' and then it could fight for such improvements as it thought necessary; and would reserve the right to take any action it thought necessary in the interests of its members.

The SMA work, at this time, included many discussions on the work of the general practitioner, of the nurse and the nursing services, and of medical service advances in other countries. The August 1947 *Bulletin* (No 90) carried an article by Dr John F. Goodall describing 'The Organization of a Group Practice' which was one of the first mentions in print of what was to develop as the private enterprise method of approaching the health centre ideal. The writer thought he and his partners had evolved 'the ideal for a group practice which can be attained by any similar group in any ordinary practice' but he made a remark which, in the light of later developments reads oddly, 'we have no appointment system (*which we believe is impossible*)'. The BMA might still be fighting for the single handed

D

practitioner but this writer and his partners had established principles 'which we think brought us success, not only financially but in making a difficult profession easy, pleasant, efficient, complete and satisfying'. The principles that produced this result were that surgeries should be designed for the comfort of the patient, every reasonable facility for investigation and treatment should be available and the doctor should do only those things for which his special training was essential, delegating other tasks to other workers.

The SMA had among its members at that time many nurses who had strong views on how the nursing services and the training of nurses could be improved. Dr Hugh Gainsborough had then a special and very active interest in this and presided over a committee set up to consider the whole subject. The Association's pamphlet *Nursing in the Post-War World* was brought up-to-date. In reviewing a report issued at this time by an official working party, Dr Gainsborough well summarized the feeling in the SMA for new thinking when he wrote 'I must bewail an opportunity lost . . . the dead hand of antiquity is still in control, and the relative times suggested for learning techniques has no relation whatever to the importance of the techniques and the sum total of the techniques represents the nursing of the past and not that of the future for which we must unashamedly plan.'

During the year the SMA renewed contacts with socialist doctors in many countries and a proposal was made to call an international conference. The International Socialist Medical Association had, of course, not met for many years but it was felt that if the SMA called a conference together, that body could be re-activated. It proved more difficult than anticipated and impossible for 1947, but from the beginning of 1948 active preparations were made and much valuable preliminary work was done.

Meantime the Minister of Health had completed his discussions with the BMA without seemingly moving the profession very much out of its original position. But much had been clarified and the profession had lost support from the public and to some extent from the Press. The Negotiating Committee had now put itself in the position that by negotiating it had in fact accepted that the new service was coming and there was, therefore, something to negotiate about. The negotiating committee actually recommended that hospital consultants should be paid by salary, which split the profession and was probably the single item which finally got the unified hospital service accepted. The consultants were at least sure of their bread and butter. Of course the Tory Party, which had voted against the second reading of the National Health Service Bill, now found it could not support, for example, the attempt by the BMA to maintain the buying and selling of practices. Above all it refused to support a body which out of self interest was prepared to defy the authority of Parliament. As the chief spokesman for the Tory Party put it, they were not prepared to support anyone who wanted 'to sabotage the will of Parliament'. It became clear as the weeks went on that the BMA was in the same position as in 1911 when it opposed National Health Insurance: it could persuade doctors up and down the country to vote its way in a plebiscite, but on the crucial day they would come into the service. The amount to be paid as compensation for the ending of buying and selling practices almost guaranteed that the profession could not stand against public opinion. Demands for speakers to explain the service poured into the SMA from every part of Britain and as the SMA *Bulletin* put it, 'What the people want the doctors will come to accept.'

May, June and July 1948 were probably the crowning months of the SMA—certainly the busiest. The Annual Conference in May occupied two busy days in which many subjects were discussed at length, health centres, nurse recruitment, control of the drug industry and so on. June was occupied with the meeting of delegates from other countries which resulted in the formation of the International Socialist Medical Association. This was held at the newly opened Beatrice Webb Memorial Home at Pasture Wood, Dorking, and was attended by seventeen delegates and observers from nine countries in addition to many SMA members. A full report was given in *MTT* Vol 6 No 7 (Autumn 1948), and we need note here no more than the fact that in spite of an enthusiastic send off the new Association failed to become a permanency. It was probably a little too soon after the war to have made this attempt for not only were the physical and financial difficulties great, but political divisions were somewhat too sharp for the compromises necessary. At any rate, the ISMA has not met again.

July was the month of the National Health Service. It was also the month of the 100th appearance of the *Bulletin* under the editorship of Dr Elizabeth Bunbury, 'a pleasant coincidence'. Dr L. T. Hilliard 'as the person who has read all the proofs' paid her a deservedly warm tribute for all the work this had meant, not only for the SMA but for the cause of health. 'It is not suggested that the NHS has come into being this month solely as a result of the efforts of the SMA, but does any member believe that it would have happened so soon and, on the whole, so satisfactorily, if there had been no organization to rally the health workers, enlighten the public and offset the BMA?' There was still a job to be done for, as *MTT* put it, the SMA had to watch the service closely as it expanded for 'its advantages must be encouraged and developed, its weaknesses must be removed'.

One subject that had not been dealt with adequately was the care of the chronic sick and the Labour Party asked the SMA to prepare a document for it on this matter. The sub-committee which considered it had the assistance of Dr Marjorie Warren who was then the accepted expert in the subject and a most important statement was prepared (*Bulletin* 103). The Labour Party also asked for documents setting out the arguments for an Industrial Medical Service and for views on the Recruitment and Training of Health Workers. For the moment everything was activity and no one suspected that the post war crisis was to hold up developments and that political change was to delay the Health Centre programme for twenty years.

Indeed 1948 finished on a note of optimism. 'The great changeover in British medicine has taken place with barely a ripple of disturbance and the gigantic new machine that will assume the responsibility for the health of all Britain's millions, replacing the old disease-treatment system with a new cooperative effort to prevent disease and improve health, has started its work.' So wrote *Medicine Today and Tomorrow* and went on to note that the BMA had issued a report on the future of Health Centres which was 'the final step in the acceptance by the medical profession of all we have advocated in these pages'. But as 1949 opened the political atmosphere was changing and the profession and other opponents of a fully socialized service were soon to find ways of preventing the rapid advance that had been expected.

The first memorandum issued in 1949 was on Medical Education and was prepared for the Public Health Advisory Committee of the Labour Party. The primary question asked was, 'How many doctors shall we train?' If the answer had been put into practice Britain might by now have enough doctors. We needed, the memorandum estimated, 'about 15,000 more doctors than we have at present' and to provide these 'we require six or eight additional medical schools'. But these new students must be educated in a quite different way. Recruited from all sections of the Community they must 'understand medicine in its social setting' and must 'realize the importance of psychological considerations and the recognition of disease in its earliest stages'. But before such views could be translated into practical terms at least twenty years were to pass and many reports on medical education to be made. A General Election was now approaching and all SMA member MPs would be faced with tough fights and a special General Election Fund was started so as to give them every aid. The SMA was now suffering from its own success. So many members were now on Boards and Committees that they could not give so much time to SMA affairs and many felt that the goal of a health service having been reached they could relax.

So, Dr Ian Gilliland, then Chairman of the Executive, was asked to prepare a document on the new tasks facing the Association and the way in which they should be tackled. This became the principal topic of the Annual Conference but there were forty resolutions touching on almost every aspect of the health service and based on what was now happening. It is strange to recall that two of the most hotly discussed resolutions were to deplore cuts already made, in less than a year, in hospital service budgets. Dr Horace Joules thought the whole hospital service was threatened by these financial restrictions and the conference agreed unanimously. The truth was, as *MTT* pointed out, that no one had realized just how poor Britain's hospitals were, and how much accumulated work had to be done after years of war time neglect (and damage). *MTT* was already drawing attention to the disparity between spending on defence and spending on health, a theme that was to recur year after year.

At this annual meeting Dr L. T. Hilliard resigned from the position of Treasurer which he had filled for so many years and endowed with qualities of treasurership quite unequalled in any organization. He had not only inspired to a large extent the increase in membership but had stabilized the Association's accounts and all the techniques of book keeping. He was succeeded by Mr Harry Barst, FRCS.

The first anniversary of the National Health Service was celebrated in a meeting at Conway Hall when over 300 attended and heard speeches by Mr Arthur Blenkinsop MP, Parliamentary Secretary to the Ministry of Health; Dr Edith Summerskill MP, Parliamentary Secretary to the Ministry of Food; and Dr A. D. D. Broughton, MP for Batley. The speakers were very frank about weaknesses, mainly due to compromises with reactionary forces, but had much that was cheering to relate. This was, in effect, the SMA's first meeting for the next General Election campaign which Mr T. C. Thomas had undertaken to organize. The Association had, however, suddenly another campaign on its hands—against the imposition of a prescription charge. As soon as it was announced the Executive Committee passed a resolution which was sent to Mr Bevan, to Mr Attlee and Sir Stafford Cripps and to the National Executive of the Labour Party. This read, 'The Executive Committee of the SMA affirms that the proposed imposition of a charge of up to one shilling for prescriptions issued under the NHS is directly opposed to the principle for which the SMA and the Labour Party have stood, namely, that the benefits of the NHS should be free at the time of use. The Association therefore urges the Prime Minister not to proceed with, and the Minister of Health to re-consider, this charge which will fall primarily on those least able to bear it.'

Meantime a pamphlet called *Anniversary Quiz* had been prepared giving many of the questions people were asking and the answers. This roused many groups to stage Brains Trust type of meetings where these and similar questions were debated. It was at this time that the Association established the practice of holding meetings just prior to and during the Labour Party Annual Conference, in the conference town, and these have remained a feature of activity ever since.

We have not noted all the deaths of prominent members during the first twenty years but toward the end of 1949 two were lost who had been exceptionally import-ant. Dr Hector Munro, a life long socialist and a founder member had been a somewhat unorthodox practi-tioner who drew his idealistic ideas from his early friendship with Keir Hardie. Major Greenwood, another founder member had been a tower of strength whenever public health and statistical studies of disease were discussed. He had a considerable influence in changing attitudes towards social epidemiology.

The beginning of 1950 was occupied with the General Election. The SMA issued an election manifesto which emphasized what had to be done to ensure 'the retention of the whole of the present National Health Service Act and its further development'. A complete restatement of SMA policy, *A Socialist Health Service* declared 'We believe that health is a right of the people, that health is an essential part of human dignity and that the health of the people is the concern of the people themselves.' The election result, it will be recalled, was in many ways a disappointment to the Labour Party but the SMA was able to congratulate eight of its members who were again returned. Somerville Hastings and Barnet Stross had very high majorities. Six members, Dr Nora Johns, Dr S. Segal, Dr S. Taylor, Dr S. Sharman, Miss C. McCall and Mr G. Drain all fought unsuccessfully. Dr Irwin Brown promptly called on the Minister of Health to recognize that as opportunity had knocked twice 'the nation and the world watch to see if the Minister will seize it with both hands'. He reminded him that 'Health is a dynamic subject and needs a positive approach.'

This article, and the SMA, fully recognized that every change in the health service that would combine efficiency with economy was to be encouraged but drew attention to an error in figures presented to the Spens Committee by the profession's 'Evidence' committee which would cost more than £2 million more than had been estimated. This point has never been corrected and in later years cost the hospital service a lot of money. The Merit Award idea, the giving of a secret bonus to certain consultants, was based on figures that were entirely false. In calculating how many specialists there were in the country, only those working in Teaching Hospitals or in voluntary hospitals were counted—about 1,700—ignoring completely some 8,000 working in municipal hospitals and other services. The Merit Award idea was accepted by Bevan because if there were only 1,700 specialists it would cost only £300,000 a year. As soon as all specialists in the country had been graded, Irwin Brown's article was proved correct but the Ministry of Health ignored it and now pays many millions for these Merit Awards. It would have been better then, and even more so in later years, if the money had been 'spent on research, on improving equipment than by arbitrarily splitting consultants into the bonus holders and the basic two thirds on whom, after all, the bulk of consultant service would rest'. The same article also calculated that a complete change from employing part time consultants to a whole time salaried service would save £12 million a year.

At the end of 1949 the Executive Committee asked Dr Ian Gilliland to undertake the work of Assistant Honorary Secretary, as Dr Bunbury had indicated she would not continue in office after the annual meeting. At that meeting in May 1950, Dr Gilliland became Honorary Secretary. Many tributes were paid to Dr Bunbury and her husband Dr Hilliard and a presentation was made to them both. They have, of course, continued their work for the Association as members of the Executive Committee, and Dr Bunbury has, with varying titles, continued to guide the Association's publishing activities and retain general editorial functions. The Association owes much to them, but Somerville Hastings paid them the tribute they probably value most when he wrote in *Bulletin* 116 (May 1950), 'it is not only for what they have done that Elizabeth and Leslie have deserved the respect and affection of us all, it is for what they have been and are —the best of friends and colleagues, always ready to listen, always ready to help. It is because they have put before all else the welfare of the organization they have so well served and because they have maintained in it the true spirit of socialism that we revere and respect them'.

The Annual Conference of 1950 had an agenda with 50 resolutions which covered every aspect of the health service. The principle resolution was moved by Dr Gilliland who gave a fighting speech on the work still to be done and on the need not only to fight for the health service but to join in the battle to create a socialist Britain. A founder member and recognized leader of the dental profession, Mr Fred Ballard, in thanking Dr Gilliland for his presentation, declared that only by the methods laid down by the SMA could the problems of the dental service be solved.

The SMA at this time took up the subject of tuberculosis with great vigour because there were still thousands of cases waiting for admission to sanatoria and yet recruitment of nurses was so poor that there were many hundreds of unstaffed beds. Dr Hugh Price became Secretary of the Tuberculosis Campaign Committee. A very important conference was held in London and many meetings arranged all over the country. In June, the Minister of Health received a deputation which pressed the Minister to launch a more active campaign to tackle this disease which was still killing nearly 400 every week in England and Wales (the great advances in chemotherapy were still to come). The Summer issue of *MTT* was given over entirely to the subject and to a full report of all the speeches made at the full day's conference. A resolution calling for an entirely new attack on the disease was passed unanimously by the 200 delegates who were present.

The Association continued its pressure on these and other points but 1951 was to bring a bigger and unexpected change which put the whole health service in jeopardy.

SIX

1951–1964

THE NEXT PERIOD of the Socialist Medical Association history need not be given in so much detail since it deals with alteration in elements of a service which was now clearly being run on the principles laid down; and the chief effort of the Association became the protection of the National Health Service from the Tory administration that was now in charge of it. Toward the end of this period when Labour came back to power it found itself facing problems which could have been dealt with during that period but which had been neglected. The greatest of these was the failure to carry out a real programme of hospital building so that by 1960 it could still be said that Britain had no example of a large modern district hospital. Between inflation and the natural escalation of hospital costs more and more money had to be found, and was found, to maintain the health service but the capital programme was neglected.

The first sign of this, it must be conceded, began while Labour was in office. Aneurin Bevan left the Ministry of Health and was replaced by Hilary Marquand. *Medicine Today and Tomorrow* saw the significance of this change which, it said, was being hailed by opponents of the national health service, as a sign that 'the revolutionary force of Aneurin Bevan appeared to have expended itself in the great effort of placing the National Health Service Act on the statute book'. What had been happening was that Bevan and his Ministry had been so busy with day-to-day administrative problems that no decisions on policy had been made in the previous year. The new Minister had therefore to recover the revolutionary spirit and make some big decisions for 'if the service does not develop it will deteriorate'—and development to *MTT* meant that 'either more money must be found or better ways of spending the health Service funds must be found'.

However, the SMA was to find itself more concerned with preserving the actual basis of the service, that it should be free at the time of use, than with getting more money than before. First the Labour Government, faced with a mounting financial crisis, imposed certain charges and 'while it is clear that constituency Labour Parties will vote against this aspect of Government policy' and while 'so delicately poised is the financial stability of the average worker that even the price of dentures essential to health or spectacles essential to industrial efficiency may be more than can be afforded', reactionaries would demand still further impositions. Indeed that was to happen within the year for Labour lost the General Election and a Tory Minister of Health brought in a charge on prescriptions which was to rouse the SMA to one of its greatest efforts.

Meantime there had been one very important change in the SMA itself. Stability among the officers had been difficult to achieve. The Honorary Secretaryship was held in turn by Dr Ian Gilliland, Mr T. C. Thomas and Dr Ida Fisher, while the position of General Secretary suffered many changes. Dr L. Ison succeeded Mr Harry Barst, who took up an appointment in the Sudan, as Honorary Treasurer. The *Bulletin* had many changes of Editor, Dr Gordon Signy holding the post for two years but it appeared spasmodically until, at the end of 1951, it was restored as part of *MTT* where it remained until at a later date that journal once again became the official journal and bulletin of the SMA.

The great change was the retirement of the President, Mr Somerville Hastings, MS, FRCS, MP. This was the 21st year of the SMA and therefore the 21st year for which he had been President and he considered the time had come to make way for someone else. No one in the Association agreed with him for he appeared as vigorous, courteous, attentive and knowledgeable as he had always done; but he was also MP for Barking, and at the age of 73 was finding all his public duties an increasing drain on his energy. The Association held a dinner in his honour in May 1951 and tried to express what he had meant to that body, to those who had known him personally, but above all what he had meant to the development of the national health service. Paying sufficient honour to such a man would be difficult in any circumstances but his own self effacing attitude, his remarkable identification of himself with any cause for which he fought, made it almost impossible to pay adequate tributes. He accepted them as he had done everything that had come his way in life, the sorrows and pleasures, as something a man had to do, for failure to do which he might be criticized, but for doing which he expected nothing.

His had been to that moment, and continued until his death in 1967, a remarkable life. His official obituaries detail his rise to consultant status as ear, nose and throat surgeon, at the Middlesex Hospital from his qualification in 1902 until his senior appointment. He was president of the Section of Otology of the Royal Society of Medicine, 1928–29 and continued at the Middlesex until his retirement in 1945. His political work is usually dated from 1923 when he won the parliamentary seat at Reading for the Labour Party but

as we have seen, his work for a national health service
had begun at least ten years before that. It was unfortunate that he lost Reading in 1924, for a continuous career in the House of Commons would greatly
have increased his influence. As it was he had to wait
till 1929 to be re-elected, lost Reading again in 1931
and did not return to Parliament until he won Barking
in 1945 with the overwhelming majority of 18,911. He
held that seat until he voluntarily gave it up in 1959. He
was thus in the House of Commons to see the triumph
of his life work when the National Health Service Act
became law in 1946. At that moment, however, his
proudest thought was that he was backed up by a team,
inside and outside Parliament, who in their own unity
of thought epitomized for him the team work he believed would change the whole course of medicine, as
indeed it has.

That team was largely his own creation. He would
himself have said that they would have come together
somehow and had the same effect sometime without
him but no one who was active in the Socialist Medical
Association over that period would agree. He was re-
markably sensitive to atmosphere and could himself
make the right response at the right moment. He had
always studied his brief, knew his agenda in every detail and was ready to guide the discussion, to reach
whatever compromise promised progress, to undertake
new responsibilities, to 'skate over the thin ice' if the
political argument was tense, or to dig his toes in if a
Minister, Labour or Tory, had to be opposed. He combined that ability to be master and servant which is the
hallmark of the first class chairman. But, above all, he
could put his ideas on paper in a logical and coherent
way—and was ready to scrap the lot or change word by
word as his committee desired. His treatment of

memoranda prepared by others was exactly the same. They were examined in the most minute detail and if needing amendment were pencilled over with suggested alterations before he came to the meeting. It must be recalled that at the same time as he was paying this meticulous attention to SMA documents he was on the London County Council, on Labour Party committees, on a great variety of other bodies, and all of them had the benefit of the same careful attention to detail. When the health service came into being he was at once ready to serve on his Regional Hospital Board, Boards of Governors and other bodies and to see in practice so much that he had visualized in theory.

To the SMA, Somerville Hastings was, of course, more than a President. He was not only a founder member but provided the young association with its first meeting place, his own home in Devonshire Street, London, and provided hospitality to innumerable and interminable committees. His wife, Bessie, played the hostess with superb simplicity serving coffee to any size of gathering, knowing everyone and what was going on but seldom offering her own opinion. No one ever had any doubt as to the support Somerville had from her in every way.

Like all busy men working for great ideas Somerville Hastings had time for many different occupations and varied interests. His greatest was in botany, particularly the botany of the garden and above all of alpine plants. He wrote many books on these subjects as he did on medical and social matters throughout his long life. His firm basic belief in the need for a national health service kept him speculating on all the different ways in which such a service could be run and it was from his speculations that others took ideas and developed them. His own words supplied much that is now part of the health service: and stimulated others to develop and put theirs into practice.

The Association now appointed Dr David Stark Murray as President and he was at once confronted with many new problems both in the SMA and in the political arena. Dr Murray was son of a former Labour MP and had been engaged in political activity all his life, and as a medical student had already become interested in the need for a state medical service. By 1951 he also had, like Hastings, the experience of seeing some of his own ideas embodied in the health service. His two war time books, *The Future of Medicine* (Penguin) and *Health for All* (Gollancz) had set out proposals similar to those propounded by the SMA. But Murray had been the first person to suggest Group Laboratories and was now in control of one of the largest and best developed, serving the hospital groups in the area of Kingston-upon-Thames. He had been one of the first pathologists to set up an 'open-access' system (1937) which made all laboratory services available to the general practitioners; and had been able to push this along under the Emergency Hospital Service and to see it incorporated in the national health service. He had a firm belief in the GP and in the need for his close contact with specialist services and provided in the laboratory regular educational meetings for all the doctors in the area. Out of these came the Kingston Medical Centre, one of the first of the modern types of educational and social centres for the combined hospital medical staff and general practitioners now an accepted part of a district hospital.

The SMA at this point took up strongly the subject of Health Centres. The Summer 1951 issue of *MTT* carried an article by Dr Peter Roe discussing the need for the rapid development of health centres especially

E

as the profession was now experimenting in group practice and was clearly becoming better prepared for health centre practice. The Autumn 1951 issue declared, 'The NHS will fail—no matter how much money is spent on it—if Health Centres are not provided.' This was an introduction to *Get the Health Centres Going Now*, a restatement by the SMA of the arguments for the immediate planning of permanent centres; but also suggesting how temporary buildings could be used and adapted. It was, however, to be many years before such a health centre programme was really to begin to provide an opportunity for 'team work' in a 'cheerful and pleasant atmosphere'. The Association was soon involved in another General Election in which the SMA Members of Parliament all had stern battles.

In previous General Elections the SMA had not only supported its own members but had provided speakers and workers in many constituencies. The main activity was in issuing leaflets for free distribution at meetings and in the 1951 election 174,000 copies of the General Election Manifesto were issued. In later elections even greater efforts were made and since then the Association has maintained a General Election fund so as to have some money ready for this purpose. The SMA contingent in the House of Commons had been reduced to six but they were still able to make their mark in any debate on health matters.

With the beginning of 1952 it was decided that although *Medicine Today and Tomorrow* should remain semi independent it should in future contain the SMA *Bulletin*, and should be published every two months, and should be of twenty pages, thus giving space for much more news of SMA work. Many meetings were organized. At one, Drs Joules, Creak and Gilliland reported on a visit they had paid to the USSR and Dr Ida Fisher delivered fraternal greetings from health workers in Rumania which she had visited. A weekend school was held at Pasture Wood on a wide programme, including international affairs. Conferences on the Chronic Sick and on Health Centres were well attended. In June a National Conference was called by the SMA Tuberculosis Campaign Committee for this disease and indeed all chest diseases, was a subject on which SMA members felt very strongly and on which, since many were Tuberculosis Officers, they could speak with great authority. They were responsible, especially in South Wales, for enlightening the miners on the subject of pneumoconiosis, with subsequent improvement in the recognition of and compensation for that disease.

At this time the SMA lost one of its pioneers, Lord Addison, who had been in large measure responsible for seeing the National Health Service Bill through the House of Lords. Christopher Addison qualified in medicine in 1891 but after a few years became more and more interested in political questions and so was elected in 1910 as a Liberal MP. During the 1914–18 war he was Minister of Munitions: and when it was decided to form a Ministry of Health in 1919 he became the first Minister. It was he who set up the Dawson Committee but before he could implement its report, lost his seat in 1922. By now he was convinced that only the Labour Party would carry out the reforms he wanted and so he stood, and was elected, as a Labour MP. In 1937 he was elevated to the peerage and so was able to assist in the passage of the bill which in some way fulfilled 'his determination to see the condition of life and health placed on a sound foundation'.

By March 1952 the SMA had a new and gigantic campaign in hand, a Petition against the Health Service charges introduced as soon as the Tories were returned to power. This was a campaign by meetings, advertisements and circularization which involved hundreds of volunteers. Nearly 90,000 petition forms were sent out and the whole country was roused. Local Labour Parties, Cooperative Political Parties, Trade Unions and SMA branches organized the collection of signatures and additional staff had to be employed to handle the petition forms. Dr Elizabeth Bunbury and the President's wife Mrs Jean Murray, undertook the office organization while Dr Barnet Stross advised on parliamentary procedures and involved as many Labour MPs as possible in this activity. Protest meetings were held all over the country. To give the Petition the greatest possible impact it was decided to make the campaign a short one, only three months, and then the Petition forms were presented to Parliament. Drs Stark Murray, L. T. Hilliard, Elizabeth Bunbury and others took the bundles of forms with 211,577 signatures to the House of Commons where they were accepted by SMA Members of Parliament, Mr Somerville Hastings, Dr A. Broughton, Dr Barnet Stross and Mr Arthur Blenkinsop. Thousands more signatures were received after that date and nearly £1,500 was received in donations to pay for the campaign. The Petition was important; but of even greater importance was the enormous response which the SMA had been able to provoke from the whole working class movement.

The SMA was thus as active as it have ever been and recruited many new members. Dr Ida Fisher and Mr T. C. Thomas were sharing the secretarial duties, Dr Gordon Signy undertook to edit the *Bulletin* and Dr Donald Degenhardt acted as secretary to a reconstituted Policy Committee. Many subjects were noted on which policy had yet to be decided. The Editor of

Medicine Today and Tomorrow took a pessimistic view of he immediate future. 'It is clear,' he wrote, 'that Health Centres, an Industrial Health Service, proper arrangements for the aged and chronic sick, a prompt attack on tuberculosis and other advances depend on he early defeat of this present Conservative Government.'

His justified pessimism arose from remarks made by he then Minister of Health, Mr Iain Macleod, at the opening of the first Health Centre, Woodbury Down, Stoke Newington. This was 'a Comprehensive Health Centre at last', and opened officially on October 14, 1952, by Mr Somerville Hastings MP, than whom 'no man in Britain could have been considered more suitable or the job'. But the Minister of Health 'tried to lessen he importance of the occasion' which was natural in a bitter opponent of the health service who suddenly found himself in charge of a socialist idea. He was not satisfied 'that the healing professions are quite sure in what sort of centre they want to work; nor do the public know in what sort of centre they would like to come to with all their different sorts of ailments'. *MTT* thought that 'implicit in his speech was the prophecy hat there are going to be very few health centres under his or any other Tory Government', but the Editor cannot then have thought that the whole Health Centre programme would be held up for more than twelve years.

For the moment the SMA had to give most of its attention to the way in which Tory Governments were harming the health service, chiefly by financial restrictions. A new pamphlet, *Hands off the Health Service* was issued and conferences and weekend schools all took up hat theme. Efforts were intensified to ensure that the Labour Party understood what was happening and

what would have to be done when Labour returned to
power. At the Annual Dinner in May 1954 the Rt Hon.
Clement Attlee MP was the guest of honour and in his
speech said he was aware 'of the many faults and
weaknesses in the present NHS but at least it was a
beginning'. The Labour Party had to regard most of
what it had done as only a first stage in reconstruction and 'intended to press forward on this framework
under the next Labour Government'.

At the Labour Party Annual Conference in the
autumn this was emphasized by Miss Margaret
Herbison who said 'a new Government would undertake to bring about better integration of the Service
and secure fairer representation on the various administrative bodies'. She also gave a firm pledge 'that Labour
on its return to power would abolish the pay-bed
system'.

The SMA had some difficulty at this time in finding
honorary officers who could give enough time to get
all the secretarial work done with the aid of the very
hardworking secretaries who were being employed. So
it was decided to appoint a General Secretary who
could lighten the work of the Honorary Secretary, and
Miss Audrey Jupp was chosen. At the annual conference
Dr Sydney Gottlieb became Honorary Secretary. By
that time the country was facing another General
Election and the SMA threw itself into the campaign.
A leaflet *Forward or Retreat?* was issued and a quarter of
a million made available to local Labour Parties. When
the Conservative Party won the election *MTT* voiced
the SMA fear that reactionary policies would mean
'medicine will be back on the market place and doctors
will be back on two standard practice, in which the
biggest purse will certainly get the quickest service even
if it does not necessarily get the best'.

During this period the SMA held many meetings on various aspects of chest disease and had a very important influence, particularly as its specialist committees on the subject had members who were recognized authorities like Dr Richard Doll, Dr Horace Joules and Dr Francis Jarman. The dramatic incident of the killing London fog of December 1952 had given the whole subject enormous publicity. The 'Clean Air and Healthy Lungs' Committee issued a most valuable report which helped to build up public interest in clean air. As the evidence of the connection with cigarette smoking and lung cancer increased the SMA led the propaganda on the subject. At the same time pressure was kept up on the subject of occupational health services but little progress was made on a programme that would be accepted by both the Labour Party and the TUC.

During 1957 the SMA Honorary Secretaryship changed again when Dr Sydney Gottlieb had to resign. His place was taken by Dr David Kerr, another general practitioner, who gave the SMA five years service before becoming an MP. Activity throughout the country was intense and a weekend school at Oxford had a better attendance than the Association had known previously, the subject of 'The Family Health Service' being of wide appeal. At the Labour Party Annual Conference the SMA meeting was crowded and two excellent policy statements on 'A New Deal for the Mentally Disordered' were made by Dr S. Sharman and Mr Arthur Blenkinsop, MP. Mental Health now became one of the Association's chief propaganda subjects, leading to important changes when next Labour was in power.

It will be readily understood that throughout its life the SMA had taken a close interest in health service developments in many countries but especially in the Soviet Union. Now there came an invitation from the Medical Workers Union of the USSR to send a delegation of SMA members both to meet the officials of that Union and to see something of the Soviet health services. *Medicine Today and Tomorrow* over the years had carried reports of visits by Dr Bunbury, Dr Len Crome and by Drs Joules, Gilliland and Signy, but this was the first suggestion of an official visit. As a result a five man delegation left for Moscow at the end of April 1958 and were back in time to report to the SMA Annual Conference. Dr D. Stark Murray led the team of Dr David Kerr, Mr T. C. Thomas, Mr H. Daile and Mr F. T. Ballard. They were received in a very friendly and generous manner and were able to give a very comprehensive report on medical care in the USSR. Above all they were able to demonstrate that medicine could cross frontiers that were still partly closed to other subjects.

The July 1957 issue (Vol 11, No 10) of *Medicine Today and Tomorrow* was a special one for it celebrated the first ten years of the NHS and 21 years of publication. A long editorial article covered much of the history we have given in these pages. Dr D. Stark Murray described the visit to Russia which was also the subject of a report by Dr David Kerr to the Annual Conference. A little later in the year Mrs Aileen Kerr and Dr John Atkins visited Rumania as guests of the Health Workers Union and reported back on the services they had seen. A year later, in May 1959, the Soviet Medical Workers Union sent a delegation to Britain and the SMA organized a programme for them. These two delegations established contact which, with occasional difficult moments, was to remain unbroken.

Once again the country faced a General Election and the SMA redoubled its efforts in favour of its members and issued nearly 300,000 of its special election leaflet. But the SMA candidates were not very successful, and Mr Somerville Hastings did not stand, so the SMA strength in the House of Commons was slightly reduced. However, the Association very quickly made its point of view clear in a resolution that the SMA adhered to 'its belief in a fully socialized Health Service unimpaired by the election results', but the fight ahead was still to be very difficult.

It was in the middle of 1960 that politics in Britain lost one of its great figures, Aneurin Bevan MP, former Minister of Health. The September issue of *Medicine Today and Tomorrow* (Vol 12, No 11) carried an appreciation of his work for health. He had, of course, made his mark in the widest of political fields but of all memorials to him, 'the greatest and most lasting will be that he saw to it that the foundations of the NHS were so well constructed as to ensure that succeeding Governments, even if they had the will, could not destroy it'. Bevan was undoubtedly a great figure for 'to have achieved greatness although a socialist and of humble origin' was not only exceptional but comprehensible only to those who shared his attitudes. He knew he was not the architect of the health service for all the sketch plans and drawings had been done over the years by many people. Bevan's greatness was that he was not the 'man to be bound by the sketch plans of any architect'. 'He had to get the building up and working not only in the shortest time but against the sabotage of vested interests.' The SMA often disagreed with him 'but never did they doubt his mastery of the subject, his determination to get the service going and his ability to make and stick by his decisions'. His biggest decision was undoubtedly his acceptance of the SMA view that 'we must have one hospital system for the whole country'. Bevan's view was, of course, coloured by his experience of the efforts of the Welsh miners to set up their own medical services. His second big decision was the abolition of the buying and selling of practices but he missed the chance to complete that part of taking medicine out of the market place by making all doctors whole time salaried officers. He could have done it, for the country was behind him, but the opposition persuaded him otherwise.

Of course, 'Nye' was accepted and admired by the working class movement for his extraordinary personal qualities. The SMA as a body had many opportunities to see him in action and to admire his knowledge of health matters in full detail and his masterly way of presenting or reporting a case. 'Everyone lost arguments with Aneurin Bevan and sometimes lost them when time has shown they would have been the better won. But no one ever felt he lost to a man who was arguing ignorantly or idly.' The Editor of *MTT* thought that one of the greatest bits of writing Bevan ever did was Clause 1 of the NHS Act, 'the first completely socialist definition of any service ever to be passed by the Houses of Parliament'.

Later he discussed this definition in his book *In Place of Fear* and gave two further versions, both typical of his own personal way of using the English language. 'A free Health Service is a triumphant example,' he said, 'of collective action and public initiative applied to a segment of society where commercial principles are seen at their worst.' He gave as examples of the triumphant collective action the supply of spectacles and hearing aids to great numbers of people who had never had a chance to see or hear properly. In the end he summarized the whole ethical, moral and socialist ideal in a memorable sentence. 'The essence of a satisfactory health service is that the rich and the poor are treated alike, that poverty is not a disability and wealth is not advantaged.'

The year 1961 must have seemed likely to be a dull one in matters of health although the new Minister of Health, Mr Enoch Powell, was trying to make encouraging noises, and the Editor of *MTT* tried to liven it up with articles for and against boxing from two labour MPs, Mrs Bessie Braddock and Dr Edith Summerskill. This was a battle which went on for a long time without either side ever having a clear cut victory.

Early in the year, to everyone's astonishment, Mr Enoch Powell not only came out in favour of developing the health service but proposed a capital programme for the rebuilding of hospitals which looked as if things might begin to move. Mr Enoch Powell was not to be in office long enough to get the programme really started but it created an atmosphere in favour of spending more money on buildings which at a later date gave Labour a good starting off point for what actually became a much bigger and better hospital building effort than Britain had ever had. The SMA, however, saw all this as no more than a façade and went on with its programme to force the NHS onwards to ever better standards. A campaign with the slogan 'Defend and Extend the NHS' was initiated, a pamphlet *Hands off the Health Service* was issued and large numbers were sold of a commemorative brochure *Aneurin Bevan*.

This new campaign made the Annual Conference of this year a very lively one. One subject that was in the forefront of discussion was the nationalization of the drug industry which the conference felt would be a better way of dealing with the high cost of drugs than by a charge on prescriptions. The Conference also passed two resolutions condemning cigarette smoking, a particularly telling speech being made by Miss Dorothy Keeling. These two subjects led to the setting up of a special committee (with Dr Horace Joules as Chairman and Mr T. C. Thomas as Secretary) to prepare evidence for the Pilkington Committee on Broadcasting. The SMA felt very strongly that advertising of tobacco and patent medicines by radio or television should be prohibited.

The SMA as we have noted had always taken a leading part in discussions about the dangers of bombing (in war time) of civilians, in the first place when high explosives and incendiaries were the weapons and then when atom bombs were used. Now it protested to both the USA and the USSR embassies about the testing of bombs which produced radio active fall-out. The SMA expressed surprise that the USSR tested such bombs within its own boundaries and appeared to ignore any hazard to its own population. The SMA, however was objecting to any and every test and demanded that the health of the world should be protected.

The Labour Party Annual Conference had not debated health questions for a year or two and probably for that reason health was given quite some time at the October 1961 conference. Dr David Kerr was the SMA delegate who moved a composite resolution on the abolition of charges in the health services and the taking into public ownership of all pharmaceutical, surgical and hospital industries. A second resolution calling for the abolition of pay-beds was also moved and many people spoke including the future Minister of

Health, Mr Kenneth Robinson, MP. The SMA composite was carried unanimously but the second was very
narrowly defeated on the plea of Mrs Bessie Braddock
MP, that the hands of future Labour Governments
should not be tied in this way.

The next two years were relatively quiet years
politically for the Tory Government had lost all
dynamism and the country was increasingly ready for
change. The SMA felt that the Labour Party was not
itself generating nearly enough energy for new policies
and at both the National Conference of Labour
Women in May 1962 and the Labour Party Conference, resolutions were put up, designed to reassert the
basic principles of the health service. These gave two of
the SMA's younger members an opportunity to put the
Association's case and to indicate that the SMA was a
force to be reckoned with in British politics. Dr Shirley
Summerskill made her first major appearance for the
SMA supporting a resolution calling for an extension of
the NHS and stressed to the women's conference the
need for Health Centres and for an Occupational
Health Service. Later in the year Dr John Dunwoody
got unanimous support from the Labour Party Annual
Conference at Brighton for a resolution mainly concerned with hospitals and indeed deploring 'the in-
adequacy of the Tory Government's ten year Hospital
Plan' and asking for increased capital spending to
replace and improve decaying hospitals.

During the year the SMA suffered two more losses.
The first, by resignation, was the loss of the General
Secretary, Miss Audrey Jupp who had given eight
years to the organization and had consolidated its work
especially with associated organizations and Trade
Unions. The second loss, by death, was a founder
member Frederick Ballard. He had been the SMA

guide in matters of dental care from the moment of its foundation and one of the most active and zestful members the Association ever had. His leadership was particularly valuable for it was based on the recognition by his own dental colleagues of his skill, integrity and knowledge. He had been a life long socialist and when he died in his eightieth year was still actively studying and advocating new ideas in dentistry.

The first weeks of 1963 were marred by the death of a younger but no less active and important member, Dr Sam Leff. Aged only 53 he was a man of such vigour, as MOH for Willesden, as a writer, as a lecturer on technical and political matters, that his death was a more than double blow. The SMA lost both a worker and an innovator who had contributed to everything the association undertook and the gap he left has never been adequately filled.

As in the previous year the SMA also had a grievous loss by resignation when Dr David Kerr ceased to be Honorary Secretary in order to devote more time to the constituency he was to fight and win in the next General Election. He had initiated many new ideas, both politically and in organization within the SMA but just because he gave so much time and energy to it he now found it was too much to be also a prospective parliamentary candidate. Dr J. Powell-Evans, a founder member took over the Honorary Secretary's post and Dr Geoffrey Richman became a very active Assistant Honorary Secretary.

At the Labour Party Conference the atmosphere reflected the rising tide of support for a change of government and Dr John Dunwoody put a resolution to the meeting which it is worth reprinting as it restated the SMA case for extending the NHS. It read:

This Conference reaffirms its adherence to the principles upon which the National Health Service was based. No development during the past fifteen years has threatened their validity. Modern medical care of the highest standard can be provided only through a service freely available at the time of need to all citizens. The defects and deficiencies of the present National Health Service arise from the failure to realize the original plan in full and the deliberate policies of the Conservative Government to refuse the money necessary to bring all services up to modern standards.

Conference calls upon the next Labour Government to bring about the full Socialist development of the service; and in particular to:

(a) remove all existing charges to the patient and return to the principle of central exchequer responsibility for the cost of the service;

(b) encourage every improvement in the status, standards and conditions of work of the family doctor, especially by the rapid establishment of health centres and the provision of open access services where they do not already exist;

(c) increase immediately the money available for the maintenance of our hospitals, giving regional boards and management committees more freedom to improve their service within global allocations;

(d) publish and implement urgently a revised ten year plan for renewal and expansion of the hospital service, providing enough beds to meet existing needs and for hospitals large enough to provide economic units especially at the level of the district general hospital;

(e) accelerate the establishment of community care services for the mentally and physically handicapped and the elderly by facilitating capital expenditure on these projects by local health authorities and by expanding rapidly the training facilities for essential non medical staff in this field;

(f) reverse the growing application of essential resources of manpower and facilities to private 'market place' medicine and abolish pay-beds from National Health Service hospitals;

(g) establish within the National Health Service at an early date a system of occupational health care;

(h) give greater attention to all measures for the prevention of ill health;

(i) devote adequate sums to research;

(j) give urgent consideration to the integration of the different sections of the National Health Service, and

(k) inspire the profession with the ideals of the National Health Service as a great social achievement still incompletely fulfilled.

There was a vigorous debate and John Dunwoody later reported that 'concern about the extent of private practice today, the importance of improving the family doctor service and dissatisfaction with the administration of the NHS were recurrent themes in the speeches'. The National Executive Committee of the Labour Party accepted all of the resolution except paragraph (f) and Mr Anthony Greenwood said that NEC 'did not believe pay-beds could be abolished overnight but were determined to stop queue jumping'. They did, however, intend to see that empty pay-beds would be fully used by NHS patients and that whenever possible amenity beds would be substituted for pay-beds. For long term planning he promised that new hospitals would have more single rooms, available for all who needed them.

The year 1964 was given over very largely to General Election matters. *Medicine Today and Tomorrow* announced that nine SMA members, of whom only three were already MPs would be fighting when the election bid came: and published messages about the part the SMA and the NHS would play in such an election, from twenty members and prominent politicians. When the election did come, four leaflets were prepared and 600,000 were distributed, a colossal effort. When the election results were announced three new SMA Members of Parliament were elected, Dr David Kerr, Dr Maurice Miller and Dr Shirley Summerskill. But the SMA had much greater support in the House of Commons for altogether 26 of its members, associate members and Honorary Vice Presidents were returned.

So it was a successful year for the SMA but marred again by resignations and, unfortunately, by deaths. Dr L. Ison, who had been Hon Treasurer for eleven years asked to be relieved and his place was taken by Miss Dorothy Keeling. The Council lost two members by death. Dr K. G. Pendse who had been for long a leader in South Wales died suddenly at a relatively early age. He was born in Baroda, India, but had been mainly educated in this country and had been from his date of qualification a GP in South Wales, much respected and a very ardent worker. Death also claimed Mr Herbert Luckett who also was one of the first and certainly the strongest of trade unionists who supported the SMA. He represented the agricultural workers and on health matters connected with the land was a very knowledgeable and helpful member: but was in every way a warm advocate of everything he thought would improve the health of the people and a firm believer in the need for cooperation between health workers and the people.

The return of a Labour Government after thirteen years of Conservative rule made this moment seem a portentious one: but with a small majority the Party had to prepare itself for fresh struggles. The SMA was now 34 years old and it too had to face internal problems and at the same time prepare policies to meet the changing political situation.

SEVEN

1965 AND THE FUTURE

THE NEXT FOUR YEARS, bringing the SMA up to its fortieth birthday should have been triumphant ones for the SMA for the Labour Party was once more in control and the way seemed open for new advances. But progress was to be disappointingly slow and there was to be another General Election before the Labour Party had real strength in the House of Commons; and this was to be followed by an international financial crisis, devaluation of the pound, and at home a threatened 'strike' by the medical profession because they were not being paid enough. But the SMA kept firmly to its task of advocating new advances and guarding the health service against inroads.

In answer to the attacks on the health service, the SMA produced *A Socialist Charter for Health* and this was made the chief subject of the Annual Conference. The President, Dr D. Stark Murray, made this the subject of his Presidential Address at the Annual Conference and tried to move the arguments that were then going on away from more money for GPs to 'a sense of collective responsibility for health on the part of the medical profession'. Embodied in a resolution which he moved was a demand 'for a sufficiently large proportion of the gross national income to ensure that the service can and will fulfil the intentions, principles and ideals of the NHS', and a statement that equally essential was the provision of health centres.

The second subject which occupied the SMA in this year was occupational health and this was the main subject of the resolution which Dr John Dunwoody moved at the Labour Party Conference. The pages of *Medicine Today and Tomorrow* reflected the growing interest in this subject which was also leading to an increase in the support the SMA was gaining from Trade Unions. The policy advocated by the SMA of an occupational health service as an integral part of the NHS, linked to Health Centres and including safety committees of the workers in every factory, gained ground rapidly and by the end of 1965 could be assumed to be the policy of both wings of the Labour Party, political and trade union.

One death saddened and yet in a way heartened, SMA members, that of Dr Henry Tabbush, MOH for Oldbury, Worcestershire. He had been a very active member in the Birmingham area for nineteen years and had contributed much to the thinking of the SMA on matters of hygiene. His death followed a long illness and what heartened other members was a letter he wrote to them all and which was delivered only after his death. While acknowledging his comradeship with those he was leaving, he still wanted to do his propaganda and asked to be remembered in a campaign advocating 'elimination of the pay-bed system'.

The President missed the General Election because he went to India for a period of six months having been awarded the first Aneurin Bevan Memorial Fellowship by the Government of India. It is of interest to recall that this had been founded by Nehru just before his death but no appointment had been made until Dr Murray was invited to accept the Fellowship. Nehru and Bevan had been warm friends and the idea was to invite British health workers to visit India and to lecture at medical schools on developments in the health and social services of the United Kingdom.

The SMA launched its usual General Election campaign and had the pleasure of welcoming two new MPs; Dr John Dunwoody and David Owen. They had even greater pleasure, as did these and all SMA members of the two houses of Parliament, when the Labour Government abolished the charges on prescriptions. Yet this was to prove one of the subjects which epitomized the difficulties the Government was to meet. The whole political atmosphere was changing rapidly and many people were moving away from earlier concepts and a whole host of movements toward fundamental changes in society, exemplified by 'student unrest', appeared to be gathering force. The SMA could not be exempt from this source of change and the Annual Conference heard an appeal for 'a campaign for a socialist society, in which health would arise from a new and better way of life'. Part of the discussion was round the title of what was now firmly the official journal of the Association, *Medicine Today and Tomorrow* and on the part it had to play in the fight for a new society and for a better health service. It was generally felt that the title was no longer valid and was finally agreed that the name should be changed to *Socialism and Health*.

This was a year of political indecision with the Labour Party losing ground in the country and the health service under constant attack. The SMA was weakened by the retirement of C. R. (Bob) Sweetingham who had been General Secretary since Miss Jupp retired five years previously. He had given very valuable service and increased the number of contacts the SMA had with the trade unions. The Association also lost its Hon Treasurer when Dorothy Keeling died at the age of 88, having been active to the end. She had long been associated with the SMA, first in the Liverpool branch and then nationally, but her work in social services had gone on for nearly seventy years. As first national organizer of Citizens' Advice Bureaux she had a national reputation but had given much time, energy and devotion to the advocacy of a national health service and then to serving within it. The SMA indebtedness to her was further increased at her death for she left a splendid legacy of £1,000 to the Association.

The year also brought the deaths of Dr Barnet Stross MP, and of Mr Somerville Hastings, the Past President. We have already noted his enormous contribution to the SMA and to the Labour Party. Dr Stross had also given many years of service, as adviser to trade unions in the Potteries, as MP, and as a Vice President of the SMA.

The continued preoccupation with health service problems at home did not prevent the SMA maintaining its interest in the development of health services abroad. Contact was maintained with the Medical Workers' Union of the USSR and in 1967 this body asked if a delegation from Britain could visit the Soviet Union as part of the celebration of the fiftieth year of the USSR. It was suggested that this should be a joint delegation with the Medical Practitioners Union and the Confederation of Health Service Employees. A full report of the visit was published in *Socialism and Health*, Sept–Oct 1967, and a number of meetings were arranged to enable the delegates to give to audiences as much information as they could about latest developments in the USSR. Provisional arrangements were made for a return delegation from the Medical Workers' Union to Britain but the troubles in Czechoslovakia caused this to be postponed until 1969. Meantime in 1968 the Hon Secretary, Dr G. Richman visited East Germany and reported back on the reception he and his wife had had from the Health Workers' Union there. Writing in *Socialism and Health* Sept–Oct 1968, on this visit, Dr Richman dealt at considerable length with the question of participation in the administrative structure by all grades of health workers. This problem appears still to be incompletely resolved in the German Democratic Republic and the SMA were intrigued when, early in 1969, they were asked to send a delegate to a conference in the USSR at which this was to be the principal subject for discussion. Dr C. R. Kenchington, who had by then succeeded Dr Richman as Hon Secretary, went to Kiev for this conference and while there opened discussions on the possibility of some Soviet doctors visiting Britain at an early date.

The Labour Party Conference in 1967 again had before it a resolution on health which was a rather omnibus affair composited from many submitted. Dr Herbert E. Bach moved it and was warmly received. In replying, Bessie Braddock MP declared for the National Executive Committee that 'no Labour Government is going to rebuild the financial barrier between the sick and medical facilities which can make them well again'.

This pledge was broken almost at once and the SMA found itself once more fighting to prevent a prescription charge. A campaign was mounted and there was no doubt of the almost universal condemnation of this tax on the sick which the SMA considered 'quite irrelevant to the economic position of the country'. Its only effect was to lower still further the prestige of a Government which, it was clear, could not be expected to carry out a socialist policy if it could so far forget the basic principles which socialists had laid down for the health service.

The death of Mr Somerville Hastings on July 7, 1967 at the age of 89 produced many obituary tokens to his work. The SMA held a memorial meeting at the House of Commons, when Dr David Kerr took the chair. The speakers, who all paid tribute to the many sides of Hastings' political work but above all to his work for health, were Lord Soper, Lady Summerskill, Tom Driberg MP, and D. Stark Murray. All of the speakers felt sure that one man who would have remained steadfast in the cause of socialism was the founder President of the Socialist Medical Association. The history of the Association was in many senses the history of Somerville Hastings for he had taken part in the struggle for a socialist health service for almost sixty years, had seen the near approach to the ideal in 1945 and had fought against every departure from the principles he and others had laid down.

He left the SMA with a firm place in the Labour Party and a job still to do. After twenty years the whole health service needed a re-examination and needed ideas if it was to become truly socialist. Approaching its fortieth birthday the Socialist Medical Association still held its place as guardian of the established service and of pioneer and guide to its future growth and development. The next years of Labour rule were to provide many happenings that justified SMA pride and many that were as frustrating as some that had occurred under Tory Governments. The continual problem arising from lack of sufficient money for all the needs of the service gave the national press the chance to keep up a constant attack on the service. In spite of annual increases in spending, in staff employed, in numbers of patients treated in new hospital building and, at last, in building Health Centres, the newspapers treated every complaint, however trivial, as evidence of 'crisis'. The impression was created of a service in decline, which was very far from the truth.

Among the complaints were many that stemmed
from the unique position of those consultants in health
service hospitals who, in order to give much of their
time to private practice, gave only part time service to
the national health service. The SMA analysed, for
example, the question of waiting lists for hospitals
admission and found evidence that these were to a large
extent a device to keep up the system whereby those
who did not want to wait could pay the consultant and
jump the queue into a hospital bed. The SMA demanded that private practice should be severed from
the national health service and consultants offered the
chance to become whole time officers, with undivided
loyalty. The Labour Party accepted this at annual conference and Mr Kenneth Robinson, then Minister of
Health, proposed a reduction in the number of private
beds but would not face up to the medical profession to
achieve the abolition of these signs of a two standard
service.

During this period the SMA also pressed on with its
advocacy of an Occupational Health Service and
showed how it could be organized as Health Centres
were built. Under Kenneth Robinson the Ministry of
Health were able to report a considerable spurt in
planning and building but when he left the department there was a slowing down of the programme.
Nevertheless enough has been done to prove in practice
all the advantages to profession and patients that
Health Centres were expected to show.

The political atmosphere, however, was full of
speculation on the future administration of the whole of
the health services, of the social services and indeed of
local government. The Ministry of Health, in 1968,
produced a Green Paper on the administration of all
health services, a document intended to provoke

discussion, which it did but met with so much opposition that when Mr Richard Crossman became Secretary of State for Health and Social Security, it was soon made clear that a new document would be necessary. The SMA put forward its own proposals which found much support in the Labour movement.

These proposals were in fact based on the principles to which the SMA had always adhered, that the form of administration should not only support but make clear, the fundamental need for a truly comprehensive service, available to all without exception and free at the time of use; but emphasized the need for a democratic structure and for the participation of all health workers in the control and development of the service. The hospital service, the SMA said, had demonstrated that health workers, as exemplified by the doctors, can play a big part in the work of all committees running the service; and this privilege must be extended to all grades of health worker. This, it declared, is an essential step to the socialization of the service and must be coupled with the democratic election of the body responsible for the day-to-day running of the service.

This insistence on the participation of the worker and the advocacy of an industrial health service brought the SMA increasing support from, and understanding within, the trade unions. The delegates of unions associated with the SMA were very active in its deliberations and made many valuable contributions to policy discussions. The greatest SMA activity was now in the industrial midlands, whereas it had formerly been in London and a combination of events led to the SMA making a move to that area, an event which concludes this history. The loss of the London office because of building changes coincided with the resignation of Dr Geoffrey Richman, as Honorary Secretary, and prompted consideration of Birmingham as a place for new headquarters. It was felt that the SMA would gain more than it would lose by working in an industrial area. Dr Richard Kenchington, a general practitioner with a long record of local political work was appointed Honorary Secretary and Mrs Joan Soan-Rethel already an Executive member, Honorary Assistant Secretary, and new offices were found.

The move coincided with the 21st Anniversary of the foundation of the National Health Service and to mark both events a conference was held in Birmingham on July 5, 1969. The President, Dr D. Stark Murray took the opportunity to summarize what had been achieved, what remained to be done and what forces had to be fought against. 'That the NHS had reached its 21st birthday, had withstood constant criticism, grumbles and complaints, had survived years of Tory rule and had expanded continually throughout these years, was a triumph for those who had inaugurated it. That it could be described by an American writer as "one of the greatest achievements of the twentieth century" was indeed a justification for all the work, thought and effort that the SMA and its pioneers had put into its foundation.'

Yet the conference ended on a forward looking note. No one now contemplated any alternative to the National Health Service: rather as international relationships improved and as the need for health services for all people became recognized throughout the world, the principles of the British Health Service were likely to become those of an increasing number of countries. The SMA was, therefore, closing one part of its history only to open another which would prove as exciting and rewarding as the first.

The ordinary work of the SMA was now accelerating.

Time was found, however, in the Autumn of 1969 to
receive a delegation from Russia led by the President
of the Medical Workers' Union, Dr Nadezhda Grig-
orieva. This visit is recorded in full in *Socialism and
Health* Jan–Feb 1970, and proved very worthwhile as a
means of cementing the tie between the SMA and the
Soviet Union. This tie is founded on the firm belief
of both the SMA and the Medical Workers' Union that
the delivery of health care must be a governmental
duty but that the standards of such a service depend on
the mutual trust and the joint efforts of health workers
and citizens. On this occasion the Russian visitors were
given a chance to make a very full assessment of British
medicine visiting Health Centres and meeting individual GPs, seeing hospitals of various kinds in London,
Birmingham, Bath, Bristol and Kingston-upon-Thames.
They also met British people from many walks of life
especially in Birmingham where they were guests at a
large Labour Club. On their last evening the London &
Home Counties Branch entertained the three Soviet
doctors and their international secretary, Mrs Natasha
Vorobieva and all were agreed it had been a memorable
visit.

The year 1970 opened with intensified discussions on
every personal social and medical service. The Government was intent on pushing through, if Parliamentary
time permitted, changes in Local Government, in the
way in which the social services are run and in the
administration of the health service. Everyone concerned with these fields was inundated with reports
and memoranda, some of very far reaching significance. For the SMA the most important was the
second Green Paper, a more exciting effort than the
first had been but very little more acceptable. It
confirmed the SMA in its belief that it was essential that

there should be a specialist body inside the Labour Party, looking after all aspects of health and endeavouring to see socialist principles more firmly applied and adhered to more strongly. It was the SMA's fortieth year, but it clearly had as much work to do to maintain the NHS as it had done in seeing it established.

INDEX